GOING
THE DISTANCE

GOING THE DISTANCE

Living a Full Life with Multiple Sclerosis and Other Debilitating Diseases

Moira Griffin

E. P. DUTTON   NEW YORK

Published in the United States by E. P. Dutton,
a division of Penguin Books USA Inc.,
2 Park Avenue, New York, N.Y. 10016.

Published simultaneously in Canada by
Fitzhenry and Whiteside, Limited, Toronto.

Library of Congress Cataloging-in-Publication Data

Griffin, Moira, 1954–
    Going the distance: living a full life with multiple sclerosis
and other debilitating diseases / by Moira Griffin. — 1st ed.
        p.   cm.
    Bibliography: p.
    ISBN 0-525-24783-1
    1. Griffin, Moira, 1954– —Health. 2. Multiple sclerosis—
Patients—United States—Biography. 3. Adjustment (Psychology)
I. Title.
RC377.G68   1989
362.1'96834'0092—dc20
[B]   89-1436
                                                            CIP

DESIGNED BY EARL TIDWELL

10 9 8 7 6 5 4 3 2 1

First Edition

For my parents

Contents

Part I

MY STORY

1

Falling

Three days a week I worked at the stable off Central Park as a lowly but self-important groom. Supposedly I was working there for the intimate knowledge of horses it would give me, but also, now that I was on my own, for the little bit of steady cash.

At five-thirty in the morning the stable was deserted except for the night watchman, the beasts (the guard dogs, the horses in their stalls, a few slinky cats), and me.

In the dark-blue morning, I'd lean against the front door waiting anxiously for José, the watchman, to let me in. While I waited, the Dobermans, who took their guarding seriously, threw themselves against the door, barking and snarling and jumping against the window to show me their impressive teeth. What sport to tear me limb from limb! they seemed to think.

Sleepy José would eventually stumble to the door and open it, and the ferocious Dobermans would recognize me and begin to grovel and wag. Menacing only a moment before, they now looked embarrassed. José disapproved of my petting them; he wanted them to be

3

nasty, which meant that they must always feel unloved. But when he wasn't looking, I'd sneak them a friendly pat.

My work as a groom was taking a toll. It was remarkably tiring. First I'd climb the ramp, slipping in the dirt and manure, humming a little tune to wake up the horses. The place would be redolent of horse sweat, piss and manure, hay and damp and dust. I'd take a deep breath, sort of a snort (which seemed appropriate there), and start turning on the lights at the end of each aisle.

The stable was gothic in the dull light, spooky as an empty church. Cobwebs crisscrossed the beams of the ceiling and a cat slithered out of my path, deserting a little pile of rodent bones, the end of her breakfast. The shadows stretched. The horses tossed their heads and rolled impatient eyes at me. They stamped: Hurry up with my hay.

At the end of the last aisle was the elevator shaft. I did that aisle first, so I could get through with it quickly. I filled two buckets with water, lugged them from stall to stall, squeezed by the big beast, and filled the trough with a splash. Then I got the wheelbarrow of oats. I tried to roll it steadily but it lurched from side to side, sloshing the oats and threatening to dump them. I scooped some into each horse's manger, then distributed chunks of hay among them. Through all this, I kept glancing at that stupid shaft. Even when I was across the room, I felt it watching, waiting, drawing me to it.

But the worst thing that shaft ever did was scare me. And give me bad dreams, although the first time I dreamed the dream called Falling, it wasn't even about the elevator shaft. That came later.

The first time, I was standing on top of a cliff. The edge was behind me. I was wearing my red shorts and my rock-climbing harness. I must have just climbed to the top because I was talking in that fast, excited, adrenaline-fired way that people do when they've just succeeded at something that deeply frightened them.

I suppose it was John, the man I had lived with, who was sitting listening among the boulders offstage and tolerating my unspeakable bravado—rock climbers and other dare-takers do this for each other. But when I turned around, laughing, and stepped into space, he wasn't able to catch me. I was already "off-belay," having unwisely untied the climber's trusty rope.

Unhitched from the umbilical rope, I fell and fell and fell like Alice down the rabbit hole. I've heard you're not supposed to do this in dreams, but I hit the bottom.

Landing in a tremendous grand plié, my five feet ten inches collapsed like a lawn chair, my knees tucked up under my chin. Then slowly, a little creekily, I stood up. I hurt. I was stiff; sort of rusty. But gradually I straightened out and was able to walk off, at first slowly and stiffly, but after a while fluidly, even jauntily.

Later on I dreamed I fell down the elevator shaft, but in my plaid flannel shirt and groom's dirty jeans. Pretty much the same story.

Most mornings at the stable, I turned on the radio. Its blare was good company and shooed away the ghosts loitering in the shadows. A sad woman sang about falling apart. That song was on the radio a lot those mornings in the late fall of 1983. The refrain was sung by a man who asked her to turn around. Turn around to what? I wondered.

By now, blue light was streaming through the window, leaving an oblong shape of the floor. The other grooms—dark men with big arms and ragged scarves tied around their heads—should have been there by six, but often they were late and I got the first horses ready for riding by myself.

Before saddling up, I'd groom a horse by going around and around on his neck, across his flanks, with the plastic currycomb in one hand—ooh, he liked that, and gave little shivers of pleasure—and a brush in the other. When I was done, he was gleaming, sleek and proud, and I stretched myself over his back and hung there like a sack or a dead man in a cowboy movie.

I could feel his heat and strength and, I thought, compassion.

Most of the school horses were headed for the glue factory when they left this stable for good. I thought that might be why their large brown eyes gazed at me with such understanding. Our best days were past; why, I was already twenty-nine. They, too, were almost finished.

I was nowhere near finished at the stable. Work didn't end until two o'clock in the afternoon. Before then, I had between ten and fifteen horses to groom and hug, ten and fifteen stalls to sweep—heavy, hard work pushing out all that wet hay and those balls of manure—and ten and fifteen little piles of sawdust to spread as clean bedding.

Just when you thought you were done, it was time to roll the drums, now full of manure and weighing who knows what, down the aisle and over to the elevator so they could be brought to street level. I think they were sold to a fertilizer manufacturer.

Rolling drums was the hardest part of the job. There was a real art to it; the sort of thing most white middle-class people never suspect. Drum rolling had been sort of a test as to whether I could become a groom or not. Some people who thought they wanted to be grooms weren't hired because they couldn't roll the drums at all. I could do it—in a fashion.

I was tall (I'm not even sure that mattered), so I could lean over the drum easily, and strong enough so I could tilt it on an edge. I'd be unlikely to let it fall on my toes (which it would have crushed). I was inordinately proud of the fact that I could, sort of, roll drums.

But I was so unrhythmic and clumsy at it. I would wobble a drum of manure down the aisle—each groom had several to do—while the other grooms stood like a row of black Mr. Cleans, looking on and smiling condescendingly. I felt desperate; they thought it was cute.

They were nice guys, though, and at times one or another would offer to help, or not even stop to offer (being clever enough to realize I'd probably resent it—although I was dying for some help) and just roll a can of mine when he had finished with his, just single-handedly roll it along, humming a little tune or something to show me how easy it was for him. Meanwhile I would gulp somebody's cold coffee and gasp, "Thank you, thank you." Then the guys would share a grin. They liked to let me know that even though I'd gone to college . . .

You had to be careful not to cut your thumbs on the ragged metal cuff inside the cans. I'd been warned over and over. Of course I sliced myself one day. Under normal circumstances seeing myself spurt blood would have made me scream and cry, but I had a certain dignity to preserve at the stable. It wouldn't do to show I had cut my thumb, so I hid it.

The next day I had a tetanus shot. New York City doctors are supposed to be unshockable, so I was gratified to see them look amazed when I said I'd been cut rolling drums of manure.

After the drum roll, it was two o'clock. My legs would be shaky and undependable by then. I'd be looking for chairs, leaning against walls, wobbling when I walked.

My tiredness exasperated me. I couldn't understand it. The work was hard, yes, but I'd been athletic since I was a kid; I thought I should be good at it. I liked to think I came equipped with a monstrous amount of strength—Athena leaping fully armored from Zeus's brow. No Venus on a half shell for me.

Being strong was a familiar buttress when my self-esteem flagged (which it was really doing those days). As I had once explained to one of my sisters, exercise was terrific because with effort, you always got better. So I thought.

I also thought I was responsible for changing (all by myself) what seemed like belittling notions of female strength. If I pooped out wouldn't the *New York Post* run headlines that no woman could handle such a tough job?

There were, of course, other women who worked at the stable from time to time who could demonstrate female competence at this stuff with much less trouble than I— but it was a handy argument so I used it during contentious inner dialogues anyhow.

All of which is just to explain why I would go riding after work even though my legs were falling off. I couldn't admit I was tired, even—maybe especially—to myself.

This was when I'd do some real falling.

Even at my best, my riding was only okay. So when I saddled up handsome and sassy Chopsticks at the end of the day, I just hoped he'd keep in mind who was on his back—the very same person who'd scratched his eyebrow bumps and fed him a carrot only hours ago—and behave.

But horses aren't like that.

Though I'd taken many horses to the park, I liked Chopsticks best. He had a rollicking canter. There was a row of magnolia trees and in the spring I liked to ride him under them—sometimes pink and white petals would scatter on us and I'd feel terribly picturesque. In the summer there might be puddles to splash through, and in the autumn dry leaves to crunch under hoof or to start at as they tumbled alarmingly across our path.

But when I'd ridden Chopsticks in the past, I had been fresh and sure, not sad, baffled by life, and tired, tired, tired.

So when Pete, a groom I palled around with, and I rode into the park that gray November afternoon, Chopsticks had a different rider astride him than when he had gone there before. I think it worried him a bit.

Not that he was bad. If I'd realized he was plotting betrayal—if he'd been really disobedient or bucked a little, for example—I might have been jerked alert. But the worst thing I could do was go along with his little rebellious pranks and act like I didn't notice—which, however, I did.

I knew my complaisance made him nervous. Just like

many people, he really wanted a boss. Someone to take charge in case anything malevolent happened.

On the other hand, maybe Chopsticks was a snob. Usually when I rode him, I was decked out in an English riding habit: skinny beige breeches with narrow black boots and a black velvet helmet. Elegant and supercilious. Arrogant and rich. Sexy but unapproachable.

Maybe he didn't like being ridden in public by a grubby groom with hay in her ponytail, a smudge on her nose, dirty jeans, and soggy sneakers. A good-looking guy like him might have been embarrassed.

I'll never know.

What I do know is that whenever Pete asked Boomer, the big gray gelding he was riding, to pick up his trot or take off into a canter, Chopsticks would be after him with a bound, no matter what *I'd* asked him for. He chased after the other horse, trying to goad him into a race. My reins would be flapping, my seat would be out of the saddle, I'd be bounced and jounced all over the place. I felt humiliated and as bewildered as a beginner.

So it was no surprise when it finally happened. Pete and Boomer were ahead of us cantering away and Chopsticks took off after them: zoom.

At first it was kind of nice. I just sat into the canter and went along for the ride. But as we went on, I began to lose my grip. My right leg seemed to grow longer and my left leg shorter and I realized I was falling.

"You okay?" Pete asked as I stood up and brushed the dirt off my jeans, smiling with chagrin. "I saw it. You just slid right off."

He had caught Chopsticks's reins as the horse bounded by him, so I didn't have to face the indignity of returning to the stable without my steed. Most of the time, when a horse dumps a rider in the park, the flustered horse goes back to the stable by himself, enters the ring, and causes a commotion, disturbing classes and so forth. When the horseless rider gets back a little later, everybody's expecting him.

But Pete had caught Chopsticks and kindly said he'd keep my slide to the ground a secret. "What happened?"

"I don't know," I said truthfully. "My legs are like spaghetti."

I was gazing at myself in the window of the subway car going back downtown and wondering who that woman was—so sad, so thin, those parentheses around her mouth, those mournful eyes . . . when a lady said, "I smell horseshit."

"My clothes!" I exclaimed guiltily. I told her about my job. I said I should have changed. She, too, became apologetic. We had to sit next to each other for fifteen awful minutes, she enduring my odor, me feigning interest in the barn behind her house when she was growing up. Finally we reached Sheridan Square, and I disembarked.

At last I was home. I ran myself a hot bath and sank into it, thinking heat would ease any soreness from the fall. But it put me into a stupor. I think I fell asleep. When I finally tried to get out, I felt like I had melted.

I hauled myself up by my arms, pushing and pulling on things—the shower curtain, the towel rod. With an odd little wooden shuffle, I stumbled into my bedroom and fell into a dead slumber. It wasn't even six o'clock.

The next day my roommate, Anna, told me to do the sensible thing: quit.

I didn't want to. Quitting the stable would be an admission of defeat; it would mean I was weak. She interrupted me: You hardly sleep, you get up in the middle of the night to go do this? It's not making you stronger, it's wearing you out. And yesterday you fell off a horse. It's a wonder you didn't break your neck.

I replied that riding motorcycles was much more dangerous than riding horses—I knew Anna liked to ride a noisy bike with some of her friends. Quite accurately she said that didn't matter.

It wasn't the only time I'd fallen off a horse in recent weeks—I'd fallen off twice in classes. The odd thing was that during the first half hour of the class, I'd do some good riding—some of my best. "Griffin, looking good!" the teacher would cry in a most gratifying way.

But then I'd lose it. Once I slid off when I was cantering around the ring in the middle of a group of horses. As I slid to the ground, I remember thinking: Well, Griffin, this is it—a hoof in the skull; you'll never be the same.

Being the fastidious creatures they are, though, none of the horses had wanted to step on the pile of human baggage. All I got was dirt in my nose and an unhappy, puzzled feeling. I consoled myself by saying all this falling was just a phase.

Maybe I did need some rest. Uncharacteristically, I told Anna she was right. Then I called the stable and said I couldn't work there anymore.

I went back to bed.

In a couple of days I felt better. I still wasn't sleeping well; too many ghosts hung out around my bed at night, playing dice and urging me to repent for some misdeed I couldn't remember. Whenever I started to fall asleep I was wakened by their laughter. They were beginning to get on my nerves.

But I had started a novel, so I worked on that a bit, as well as on a directory for lawyers and my thesis for a master's in journalism. And I went to the gym.

I had met Anna in the gym. We both stood out there—not too many of the women worked out the way we did, though, unlike me, Anna was really a bodybuilder.

I loudly proclaimed that weight training for strength, which was what I said I did, was one thing; but weight training for "aesthetics," as Anna called looks, was another—was, well, *vain*. Contests of physique were embarrassing displays of narcissism, I contended.

Anna wasn't fooled, though. She gleefully acknowledged that she wanted to be "cut" (have sharp muscle definition) and had piles of magazines featuring women bodybuilders with skimpy bikinis and oily flesh. Often she'd curl up her arms to show me her biceps or roll up her shirt to show me her ridgy abdominals.

I hope we don't sound like two Valkyries trying to outdo each other—we were more like neurotic beauty queens. Anna was tiny—five foot three and one hundred pounds, blonde and pretty (though the studded belts and black leather were a bit unsettling). And though I was more than half a foot taller, I was hardly a bulldozer.

Anna's life-style didn't appeal to me. It was rigidly organized into working out and going out—which usually meant dancing until dawn somewhere in this big city. After working all day as a secretary at the university where she was finishing an advanced degree, she went to the gym, came home and ate her fish and salad, and went to bed for a few hours. At ten she rose again and put on her fishnet stockings and black leather miniskirt and took off for the night.

Okay, so it wasn't the life for bookish me. I still thought she had the courage of her convictions.

Anna ran five miles every morning. So what?—I'd work back up to six. I knew I was a better swimmer, so I swam a mile a day on top of running. And of course I worked out at the gym—mostly because I liked it, but also because I didn't want her to get ahead of me there.

I continued the directory and the novel, even did a few little free-lance jobs like proofreading, but most of the time I spent exhausting myself. Giving up the stable work didn't give me more rest—I just stopped getting paid for pushing myself to the limit.

Yes, the one-upmanship was petty and is embarrassing to contemplate now. I felt inferior to Anna—she was pretty and dramatic and smart. She was deliriously in love, while I felt bereft, used up, unlovable. And she was threatening my very dear self-image as the most athletic woman I knew. So who was I? If I wasn't part of the couple I'd been with John, and I wasn't this exceptionally athletic woman . . .

Then I thought about a triathlon.

A triathlon! What a way to show what I was made of. I went to a sporting goods shop and bought a magazine that had a list of upcoming triathlons in the back. There was a picture of a female champion on the cover, which I tore off and pinned to my wall for inspiration.

I bought a bunch of little notebooks to log my training in, read the magazine, and planned a workout schedule. I figured it would take ten months or so to make a triathlete out of me. I wanted to do just one triathlon—and now I had the time to train for it. After doing one, I figured I'd get a regular job and use my evenings to write. I put the current novel and its outline in a typing paper box, thinking it would wait for me.

I was in training.

I got up in the morning, had a cup of tea, and went into the living room to do my crunches (modified sit-ups) and what I called tilts—Jane Fonda's suggestive exercise for the buttocks. Then I ate a bagel and went out to run.

This was the best moment all day: stretching out my legs and circling Washington Square in sloppy gray sweat pants and a turtleneck jersey. The air was brisk and clean, the sky hard and gray, my strides long and exhilarated.

But something odd began to happen. After only a few times around the square, it became difficult to lift my knees in a running gait. My right foot misbehaved, hitting the ground flat-footedly. Slap, slap.

I started to weave. I finished the three miles, but it was as if I'd gone much much farther. I was unsteady on my feet, every step unsure.

Maybe I was overtraining. Instead of running every day, I'd run every other day, for starters.

The tiredness and wobbliness weren't all that began to happen, but they were all I paid attention to. The other things I experienced were even stranger. I didn't know what to think about them, so I didn't think about them at all. For example, the ground began to wave. It would swell and billow under my feet, even if I was standing on concrete; as if I were on a boat rocking back and forth.

And my body always seemed to be a few beats behind my mind—for example, I'd think *Stop* when I got to a curb but my legs would take another couple of steps of their own accord before they got the message. I'd be in the middle of the street with New York City traffic hurtling toward me. I kept bumping into people who, in true New Yorker fashion, glowered at me.

Worst of all, though, I was so emotional. I'd cry torrentially at the slightest provocation—even without provocation. I had fights with everyone. And I had religious thoughts—for an unbeliever, a bizarre experience.

Scenes from the Bible that I hadn't thought about since parochial school twenty years ago filled my mind. One in particular: Jesus in the Garden of Gethsemane asking his Father to "let this cup pass," meaning the suffering to come.

But despite these daydreams and the billowing sidewalk, it wasn't until I fell flat on my face that I let myself realize that something was wrong. Looking back, it's obvious that a lot was wrong—I was very depressed, as well as physically sick. But I didn't think so then. I thought depressed people refused to get out of bed or wash their hair in the morning, whereas I was so *active* and not only washed my hair but wore mascara every day, even when I was working at the stable (do you think the horses noticed?).

But one day I fell. It was my fourth time running around Washington Square. I saw this wet yellow leaf in the middle of the sidewalk. I ran on it, it slid a little, I hit the pavement.

I got up and tried to resume running, but it was as if I were moving through quicksand. I grabbed a traffic signpost to steady me. Actually, to hold me up.

The uneasy feeling lurking inside me had me by the shoulders now and was shaking me, shouting "There's something wrong with you, really wrong!"

I held on to the signpost, feeling dazed. *Really* wrong? Something *bad*? Could this be?

Instead of trying to finish the three miles, I went

home slowly, up lower Fifth Avenue past hordes of laughing NYU students. This time I paid attention—I was wobbling, wasn't I? Staggering like a drunk. Half jokingly, I told myself to prove that I was sober, I'd walk that line in the sidewalk.

First I lurched two steps to the right and then I corrected it and lurched two steps to the left. I tried again. And again. Carefully now, concentrating and taking it easy, I tried again.

2

Finding Out

When I woke up the next morning, I knew I had to see a doctor. Soon.

I went through the motions of normalcy, putting on heels instead of sneakers though, since I was meeting Cynthia, my older sister, for a fancy lunch at noon. Affectionately fussy, Cynthia often scolded me for being too thin. I was already on my way to meet her when it occurred to me that I *was* terribly thin, so I stepped into a coffee shop and ordered a bowl of minestrone soup.

Not that soup would fatten me up in half an hour, but I had to have something fast or I'd have no answer when she said reproachfully, "What have you eaten today?" Dutifully, joylessly, I ate the crackers, too. How odd my wrists looked, so white and sharp, out of my coat. Whittled bone.

I left the coffee shop and walked down the street crying. If I ducked my head maybe nobody would notice. I couldn't stop; tears squeezed out of my eyes and rolled down my cheeks.

Something was wrong.

Cynthia was prompt as usual, waiting for me outside Bloomingdale's. "You're very thin," she said. She was wearing bright turquoise, with something expensive and furry; she looked pretty, shiny, and brand new. Like a Christmas toy, I thought with the resentment of unresolved sibling rivalry.

"Something is wrong with me. It's worse than missing a button for an eye!" I shouted suddenly and incomprehensibly. (I think I meant I felt like an old toy, maybe a stuffed bear, who had lost its button eye.)

Cynthia stopped in the middle of the busy sidewalk and looked at me gravely. "Nonsense," she said.

We went to a dark Chinese restaurant. Over the egg foo yung I tried to tell Cynthia that something really was wrong. I wanted to see a neurologist—they were awfully expensive but I had to, I said wildly. Could I borrow some money?

Instead of answering that right away, Cynthia scolded me. In her best big-sister, I've-been-through-it-all-before-you voice, she told me that nothing was more painful than the end of a love affair. Years earlier, before she'd married, an unhappy ending to a love affair had made her physically ill, she said. "Eat some egg foo yung, it's nutritious."

I thought she was missing the point and squirmed with impatience. First of all, living with John was not just a "love affair," I told her huffily. Almost seven years! Nor were these physical symptoms the usual sort of misery that follows a romantic disappointment.

Cynthia answered calmly. She said she had a friend who was a psychiatrist at Metropolitan Hospital and would know a neurologist there, if I really thought I needed one. "But," she added, "if you stop crying, you won't choke on the food so much." And the reason I staggered that way when I got up was because I was upset. But as we were leaving she said that I was not to worry about the doctor's bill; she'd take care of it.

I called her friend as soon as I got home. Sitting hunched up on my bed, I curled around the phone while her friend gave me the third degree. I said I had fallen and that I often wobbled when I walked—I told her about the crack in the sidewalk. She asked if I was taking drugs. No. Was I drinking? No! Rather, a little once in a while, but moderately. She asked about cold capsules, any medications. Then she abruptly said okay, good-bye.

Cynthia called me later. Her friend had given her the name of a smart neurologist at the hospital. She said if I was having trouble walking, it should be taken seriously.

So. See? I wasn't crazy. I *should* be taken seriously.

Now I was really scared.

The neurologist's office at Metropolitan Hospital was very white. The couches looked like snowed hedges or maybe snowed cars. I wondered why Cynthia had insisted on coming with me. She looked so out of place in all her colors, perching on the snow like some gorgeous tropical bird. I was glad she was there.

But she was there only to humor me, right?

For the first time in a doctor's office, I didn't have to wait. He wanted to see me all too soon.

The neurologist was a little guy with a big Indian name. "Walk down the hallway," he said, so I did, thinking I was doing pretty well, thinking I wasn't wobbling at all, although I guess I was a bit. I was concentrating with all my might and going a little more quickly than necessary—the momentum might help me stay straight, I thought.

Though I'd wanted to see him so much, I was trying to hide my symptoms. It was a lot easier to talk about my odd problems than to *show* them—there was something shameful about my body being out of control. Words, talking, writing were my way of being in control, even when being out of control was the subject. I wanted to *tell* him, not show him.

But "Stand on your toes," he said, after my walk down the hallway.

"I'm not very good at this," I said apologetically.

This was so simple yet so impossible. I used to dance *en pointe;* remember my enviable arabesque? Now, standing on my toes seemed rather daring. I might topple over, I thought.

I did well at the strength tests. He took my hand and said, "Pull me toward you," and I pulled him right into the table. "Umph. You're strong as an ox," he said, straightening his white coat. And since I couldn't do all the things he told me to do, like walk heel to toe in a straight line, I started feeling mean—not even sorry if I hurt him a little when he collided with the table. He said, "Lie down, please," so I lay down, crinkling the paper on the white table. I lifted my legs straight up and he tried to push them around but I was steadfast—oh, no, you won't! My legs in my nice corduroys stayed straight up. (Well, almost.)

Then he took a pin out of his pocket and traced little circles on my belly with it. I caught a strange look on his face as I calmly watched him. "Do you feel this?"

"Yes, it hurts—are you done?" I tried to sound jocular, though neither of us was fooled. How am I supposed to react to this pin on my smooth stomach? I wished somebody would tell me, but nobody would. He kept making circles with the pin. We both watched him.

"Please stand with your feet together and your eyes closed again."

Ah, this is difficult—what sways like this, bamboo?

"You're swaying," he said.

Yes, there's a gale wind, I thought.

Then eye tests. We both sat down and he smiled, but he had one more awful task. Count backward by sevens.

He thinks there is something wrong with my mind! Mentally I whirled in a vortex and said, "No. I won't count backward by sevens. No."

He looked at me oddly and sympathetically. He feels sorry for me! Why, what does he know?

"Do you think you have a brain tumor?" he said quietly.

Although I was sure I hadn't thought of this before I heard myself gasping, "How do you know?"

"I don't know. In fact, I don't think so. But let's get you a CAT scan right away."

Ah, more to humor me, the anxious patient, I said to myself, not thinking about counting backward, not thinking about why he might want a CAT scan if not to humor me. Well, I am being taken seriously here, but I don't like it. This is becoming very expensive; why does he think I need to be humored this much? Why is he taking this *so* seriously?

But I meekly went down the corridors of Metropolitan Hospital and into a room where three technicians waited by a space-age machine. So I'm going to be doing some time-traveling, I thought.

I lay down in the time-travel machine, hoping a better life awaited in the other dimension. The technicians strapped me in and warned me not to move my head when the machine started up, and a heavy blonde with dark roots leaned over me and said she was going to put dye in my veins.

But this woman whose name was Carol had a hard time getting the dye into my veins. She stuck me with the needle and then yelled, "It's blowing!" I was strapped down and couldn't see what was blowing. She tried again with a new vial of dye and still couldn't get it, so she tried the other arm. After her fourth poke I lifted my head and asked, "How many times are you going to try?"

Someone had already called a doctor to help me and the miserable Carol. The young male resident was soothing. He told me to bend my elbow and pump my arm a little. When he saw my biceps bulge he said, "Are you on steroids?" This made me like him; I thought he was admiring my slender but curvacious arm and that he was talking about anabolic steroids, the kind muscle men use to beef themselves up. But probably not. Most likely he meant corticosteroids; I found out what they were later.

Mistaken or not, I was flattered so I laughed and began to flirt a little, as well as one can when lying strapped into a CAT scan. He easily pricked my arm and the dye rushed in. "You're going to feel very warm," he said, and smiled, while I felt a warm rush through my body, down to my toes and centering in my crotch.

"Well, it's not unpleasant." I smiled back and batted my eyelashes.

The good young doctor laughed amiably and gave me a reassuring pat on the shoulder, which made my face crumple briefly. He disappeared and the platform I was on began to slide into the doughnut hole of the CAT scan while all the technicians hid in the other room from the X rays the machine was emitting.

They forgot to cover me with the lead blanket. Only my head was supposed to be irradiated. I bent my head up and glared at them staring at me from behind glass in the observation room; then I stared at the blanket at my feet.

I thought this primitive communication was successful but nobody wanted to come out—how dangerous were these rays? Finally the girl who got the doctor ran out and hurriedly pulled the lead blanket up to my chin. The platform I was on moved another few inches into the doughnut-shaped opening. It stayed there a few moments while that section of my brain got x-rayed, then moved a little farther in.

That's all. The technicians unstrapped me and I got up on shaky legs and hurried into the adjacent room where Cynthia was waiting, reading an old magazine. I fell to my knees like the heroine in a melodrama and while I was crying and trying to tell Cynthia about Carol poking my arm over and over and screaming It's blowing! a nurse asked kindly if she could get me a glass of water.

I realized then that I was exaggerating, and started to laugh. Cynthia seemed to think I'd been tortured. We went back upstairs and sat in the white room.

Pretty soon the doctor called us. He sat me on a table while they both sat on low chairs. I saw through this manipulation (he was trying to make me feel powerful by seating me above them—nice of him), yet I was only mildly abashed taking the highest seat. I knew he was right—I was so frightened, I needed it. He had the CAT scan photos in his hand.

"Well, you don't have a brain tumor and you haven't had a stroke," he said triumphantly.

Of course not, I told myself. It was silly of him to think I might have. "And I see no reason to think this is psychological," he added, a remark I found mysterious. Who would imagine this could be psychological? "But we have to do further tests before starting any treatment."

I wondered why he thought I needed treatment. I just need to sleep more, take it easy, I wanted to tell him. There's nothing wrong with me, not really.

We made an appointment for further tests, "evoked potentials" this time. I had no idea what those were. "They don't hurt," he said, "but be ready to spend a whole day here." Before we left I asked the million-dollar question: "What do you think is wrong with me?"

"A virus or an allergen," he answered promptly. I naïvely thought these were innocuous.

The doctor followed me out of his office and whispered teasingly, "Can you count backward by seven?"

"Ninety-three, eighty-six, seventy-nine, seventy-two, sixty-five . . ."

"I thought so," he said, and tapped me with the file he was holding. We both laughed.

What a nice man. I was sure he was taking this all too seriously, but after all, that was his job.

The evoked-potentials day came soon. This time my three sisters were with me—Cynthia, Regina, and Becky. Cynthia insisted on being there (not that the protest I made was genuine) so I guess she asked Gina and Becky to keep her company. But it seemed a little odd; these trips to the hospital were becoming a family excursion. The four of us had fun on the way though, telling stories and laughing uproariously, the way the Griffin girls always do.

The part of the hospital where the evoked potentials were done was grim. The walls were a bilious color and there was no waiting room for my sisters, just three plastic chairs in the hallway.

This time Cynthia let me act as if I knew what I was doing, so I followed the nurses into the office alone and tried not to look horrified when they said I had to pay up front—$700! None of it was covered by my paltry insurance. I wrote the check knowing my account wouldn't cover it, but that my big sister would deposit enough into my account to pay it.

Why didn't anybody tell me about the costs? I wondered. I felt babyish, belittled. You need money in the adult world, and I didn't have it. My romantic notion of being an artist and amateur athlete began to look stupid. That's a fiction, I berated myself. You idiotic, incompetent baby! I felt the first wave wash over my head.

I followed the technician into a dim green room where several machines waited. They looked like television sets. She talked a mile a minute about her own life while she sat me down in front of one and scratched several places on my head, then taped wires to those places and turned the machine on.

"Keep your eyes on the middle of the screen," she said. It was a checkerboard so there was a square there but then the screen began to bulge and move. I couldn't help but let my eyes follow the trajectory of some of the flashing squares. "Keep your eyes on the middle!" she scolded.

She's not looking at me, but I think she can tell I'm not keeping my eyes still by the zigzags on her screen. Are those my brain waves? I wondered. Oh, my secret wrongness is out! I'm mad at my brain for letting the mistakes it's making show up on her screen—now everyone will know!

Then we did auditory evoked potentials. She put headphones on me, and I heard a soughing as in seashells. Maybe banshees sound that way. But that wasn't the noise she was asking about. Soon I heard various beeps and blips—that's it, she said—and I obligingly moved my fingers to show her how long they continued.

By then it was afternoon. She offered me a piece of candy and asked how I felt. "Bored," I answered, which made her laugh.

"Good thing you didn't say it hurts," she said. "There's nothing I can do about that. This is the last test. Do you want another piece of candy?"

I do, I do. I want an Easter basket full of chocolate eggs. I want a white horse, a milk-white steed. I'd name him Neptune and he'd carry me away over the sea.

"Okay," I said.

She gave me another piece of hard candy and I got up on another white table. She scratched my head and my back, taping lots of wires onto me this time for the soma evoked potentials. I lay down. She started the machine. My leg hopped.

Wow! I sat bolt upright, tearing out all the wires that were attached to me. "My leg hopped!—I didn't tell it to," I said. She laughed and told me that a harmless electrical impulse flows from the machine down the wire and into my nerve telling my leg to jump like that. "I want to watch," I said, so she used longer wires to let me sit up and watch as the electrical impulses made my leg jump around, totally without volition. Weird.

Out in the hall my faithful sisters waited for me. By the time I was done, they were famished. I was excited about the soma evoked potentials but they looked at me as if I were nuts—that was *fun*? "No, but interesting," I said, wondering about nerve impulses and electricity, and what "evoked potentials" meant.

The next day Anna, brushing her hair before the bathroom mirror, said, "Even if it is multiple sclerosis, that's not necessarily so bad, you know."

"What?"

"Let's not write the script," she said.

Multiple sclerosis, multiple sclerosis, a chorus of unfriendly voices hissed and gurgled.

What made her think it was MS? I didn't dare ask. Anna knew a lot about diseases, since she was a hypochondriac. Maybe she knew why they gave me those bewildering tests. I shuffled into my room and picked up the dictionary by the bed.

"Multiple sclerosis. A chronic progressive disease in which patches of tissue harden in the brain or spinal cord, causing complete or partial paralysis," said my *Oxford American Dictionary*.

My back stiffened, grew spiny as coral.

I sat there awhile, then tried to call the neurologist. "Do you think it's multiple sclerosis?" I practiced saying while I waited for someone to answer his phone. But I hung up when I heard his receptionist's voice.

There wasn't enough oxygen in my room. I tried his number again but hung up again. Finally I called Cynthia.

"Maybe it's multiple sclerosis," I said. "Would you call the doctor and find out? I can't."

Cynthia called back in fifteen minutes. "He wants to see you again and says he'll have a diagnosis then. We have an appointment for January sixteenth." So I have to wait until after Christmas, I thought. I have to wait until 1984.

There was snow on the ground in Connecticut when I went home for Christmas and an air of unreality about everything I did. I remember being careful and rather polite with myself as if I didn't know me, as if I were a stranger.

Fear of slipping on the steps leading out of my house made me clutch the railing, creeping slowly. An incriminating path of footprints made a big uneven arc in the snow when I staggered to the car.

"I'm tired," I said to my staring family as I fell into the car's backseat.

"You had too much egg nog," joked my father, though we all knew that wasn't true.

For the first time in years my father didn't shake his head and mutter "Speedy Gonzalez" as I bounded up the stairs of the house where I grew up. I used to take them two at a time, but I held the railing that year, climbing them cautiously.

I'd already broken a finger when I fell off a stepladder reaching for a book on a high shelf. A rock climber won't fall off a stepladder, I had told myself as I climbed the steps, laughing at the odd feeling of insecurity I had, the feeling that I was ignoring some important warning. Then I reached up for the book and fell. The old rules didn't apply anymore. I gripped the railing and took the stairs seriously, wondering if they could be as difficult as they seemed.

Christmas passed. Inexplicably I forgot I might be an invalid and was seized by a great desire to ride a horse. I called the stable where I'd fallen off at Thanksgiving.

"I want a class," I said. "I want to jump."

Right after New Year's, Regina and I drove into the Connecticut countryside, leaving the car at the bottom of the hill and trudging through drifts of snow to the sprawling white stable. The horses were blowing jets of steam through their nostrils and I found my name on a bulletin board next to that of Geronimo, the horse I was going to ride. So I tacked him up, made friends with him, and led him to the ring in the other building.

The teacher was waiting for me there, stamping her feet and blowing on her fingers. Geronimo and I felt frisky, and we cantered around the ring a few times—so easily, so fluidly—before stopping before her and listening politely while she pointed out the course of fences we should take. We sailed over them—one, two, three, four—let's do it again, though she didn't say to—one, two, three . . .

"A breakthrough! A breakthrough!" shouted the teacher, raising a brown cloud around her stamping feet. "A breakthrough!"

This was fun. Geronimo and I went around again. Sometimes you need a little break, I thought, stopping in front of the teacher and doing a little dressage dance for her.

"Great," she said, and made the fences higher.

"Let's show her how it's done," I said to Geronimo. We took the heightened fences with no problems. Regina, watching from the bleachers, clapped.

The hour went by fast. But when I slid down the side of Geronimo, I found I had to keep holding on to him to stay standing up. I hoped Regina and the teacher didn't notice. Nonchalantly I gripped the saddlehorn with both hands and let them think I was petting the horse. "Walk him down," the teacher said, and went into the office for a mug of hot chocolate.

So my horse and I walked slowly around the ring until we stopped sweating. Amazing how quickly one got out of shape, I thought. It was the best jumping I had ever done, but when I first slid off I had felt so weak.

The next day I went back to New York.

January sixteenth was the date of my appointment with the neurologist. I was amazed to see Cynthia, Regina, Becky, *and* my mother sitting in the waiting room when I arrived, only a few minutes late.

"I've got a retinue today," I said to the neurologist, who was waiting for me, too.

He didn't smile. A little vein pulsed in his jaw.

I watched the vein and the set mouth. Oh, no, I thought. Oh, no. He's got bad news.

I followed him into his office and took a chair across the big important desk from him. He shuffled some papers, then stacked them on the desktop.

He started by telling me about the blood tests and the terrible things that I didn't have. Then he said he had also received the results of the evoked potentials.

"Well," he said.

"Yes," I said.

"There are, um, abnormalities," he said.

"Oh," I said.

Then he told me that something was wrong with my vision (but my eyesight had always been excellent!) and something was wrong with my audition (but my hearing had always been good!). Something was wrong with my sense of position—my brain received messages from my body a bit too slowly, so I couldn't react to the information in time. It was something I wouldn't even notice, except that the slowed transmission of messages about body position was why I couldn't keep my balance as I used to.

I looked away from him at my very nice new shoes.

"We'll have to call this multiple sclerosis," he said.

I was wearing very nice new shoes. Off in the distance to my right, a small voice was telling me something about platelets, and that he wasn't an expert in MS but concentrated on venous problems, or stroke. After contemplating my shoes awhile, I turned back to this very small man across this wide, wide table, and said, "What?"

"MS," he said.

I looked back at my shoes.

After a while I began to cry and he stopped talking. I sobbed and sobbed, then abruptly looked up and said, "What can I do?"

"Almost anything—I mean, anything that you can do."

"I mean: What can I do to get better?"

He hung his head.

I stared at the top of his head a moment, then sobbed some more. When I looked up he was still staring at the desk. I said, "Look, I know there's no cure. But isn't there something I can do?"

He brightened. "Have a good attitude," he said.

I laughed crudely.

"And see a psychologist."

"A shrink! How's that going to help?"

"It will help you cope."

"Cope? Cope! *I'll* cope," I said with characteristic bravado. "How can a shrink help me cope?"

The neurologist didn't answer, and I cried some more.

3

Reeling

I lay on Cynthia's big white bed during the day and considered how unfair, how wicked, it was that this should happen to me.

Alone in her room, I screamed that I didn't deserve MS. Over and over my rational self answered: *Deserve* has nothing to do with it. I wanted passionately to blame someone. If I had *deserved* it, I could have blamed myself. In a deep and irrational way, I did.

Most of the time I spent absorbed in grief and guilt and fury. Somewhere in the past I had done something so evil that I couldn't even imagine it now, and the God I claimed not to believe in was taking retribution. What had I done? Why hadn't I been told the cost? Cruel God, just tell me how and I'll undo it.

I wanted vengeance, too. If God was behind this, I wanted to make him pay.

After a couple of hours I'd get tired of this—for awhile. I knew it was irrational and that I was being vicious to myself, so I watched funny movies on Cynthia's videocassette recorder. Cynthia had read Norman

Cousins's *Anatomy of an Illness,* and advised me to laugh as much as possible. Cousins thought laughter had helped him beat a serious illness. Although I thought this sounded dubious, I figured it couldn't hurt.

I spent most of the day in bed because when I got up, I felt as if a walnut were rattling around in my skull. This feeling—like the most excruciating hangover—was the result of the spinal tap I'd had to confirm the diagnosis. Though only a small amount of CSF (cerebrospinal fluid, the cushioning stuff the brain floats in) had been taken for testing, I imagined the remaining fluid ran down my spinal cord, which I pictured as the hollow tail of the brain, when I was upright, leaving my brain without its cushion. So I lay down to keep my brain afloat.

But I doubted if all this lying down was good for me. On the one hand, I needed the down time to register the new information, to learn to bear the feelings. It would have been like me to avoid them by doing things—until recently, by exercising furiously. But lying flat on my back, I could avoid the feelings only temporarily—and avoiding them temporarily was in order, since they were so intense—before there was nothing to do but confront them again. Occasionally turning on a funny movie was like coming up for air before sinking back into the angry ocean. The sinking was as important as the coming up for air, because knowing how you feel is the first step toward feeling better.

On the other hand, being able to do nothing for a while gave me the idea that I was worse off than I really was.

I had started going into remission around New Year's, apparently—that would explain why I was able to ride Geronimo so well. The exacerbation—the few weeks when the symptoms had been most evident—had not been dramatic. And it had ebbed already. But I didn't know how far it had ebbed. And I couldn't know—no one could know—how long it would stay that way.

•

I was living with John again. I had called him at work from Cynthia's after the doctor gave me the grim verdict, and told him my bad news.

"May I stay with you tonight? I don't want to go back to Fifth Street; I don't want to sleep alone."

"Of course," he said.

John and I had stayed close after I moved out. He called me several times a week when I was rooming with Anna, just to talk. There was an emotional dependence on both sides.

During the week following the diagnosis and spinal tap, I shuttled between Cynthia's apartment during the day and John's loft at night, lying down in the backseats of cabs. During one of my cab rides, I was lying on the backseat and I started sobbing. After a few moments the cab driver, a white-haired man with a middle European accent, pulled over to the curb. "You're a good person," he told me earnestly. "A good person."

"But I'm sick," I said, as if that proved him wrong. "And I'm not going to get better," I wailed. (This was unfair—he probably thought I meant I was dying. MS, however, is very rarely fatal. Most people get to live with it for a long, long time.)

The cab driver finally dropped me off at Cynthia's and reminded me again that I was a good person. His old face, homely as a potato, watched me hurry into the chic Upper East Side building. I felt embarrassed, partly because I had broken down in front of a stranger and partly because I had led him to think it was worse than it was. I also felt grateful for his concern. He didn't have the vaguest idea who I was.

Lying down so much that week made me fidgety. Cynthia had a copy of Jane Fonda's videocassette workout and I decided I wanted to watch that, even if I couldn't jump around with Jane. The tape showed strain and zeal and gasping for breath. I missed that sort of thing.

I stuck the cassette in the VCR and lay down on the bed to watch other people exercise.

Jane was so gung-ho. Suddenly I felt angry. I had always assumed that forty-five would find me energetic and shapely, too. But now it seemed that this was not to be. Somehow I felt she was pitying me or taunting me or both. Finally she got to the push-up part of the tape. She bent her knees. Ha!

I could do push-ups, I thought. I could do real straight-leg push-ups, tougher than the kind Jane was doing. I'd be nearly horizontal through the whole exercise, so my head would be okay. I got down on the floor and began puffing and pushing away.

Just then Cynthia came in. She shook her head. I can't blame her, but at the time I had to do these push-ups.

"Humpty Dumpty sat on the wall, Humpty Dumpty had a great fall. All the king's horses, and all the king's men, couldn't put Humpty together again."

I was on my way to the stable, a few weeks after the diagnosis, reciting that nursery rhyme under my breath, like any other New York City crazy. The spinal tap headache was gone and I thought I should waste no time before getting back into the saddle (literally). I felt defiant: Nothing's going to stop me.

At the stable I asked for an old war-horse named Legend. He was big and clunky and I thought he'd be good to ride on a day when I wanted a horse that didn't demand much of its rider.

However, he was not only old but wise.

He must have smelled fear on me—I was very afraid of life in those days. (How does fear smell? Sour, I think, like a lemon. Maybe that's where we get the phrase "He was yellow" to describe a coward.) In any case, Legend didn't feel safe with me. He wouldn't trust me, even in the indoor ring. I sat securely in the saddle and urged him forward with my heels. But Legend wouldn't budge.

Then I tapped him with my stick. He stayed recalcitrant. I hit him harder: Nothing.

At last I slid off and led him to the ramp where he moved very fast.

"I don't know what's wrong," I lied to the riding teachers. "Legend refused."

We called another horse, a fast, excited, long-maned mare, Caramba. She was rearing to go. She sensed my fear, too, but it made her move faster. I had to hold her back.

When I got off I was exhausted and shaken. I kept thinking about Legend, who wouldn't take a step for me, and the mare who wanted to run away. I knew they sensed disaster. Maybe they knew what was going to happen.

In John's loft there were two poles or columns between ceiling and floor. Several times a day I worked on my balance by trying to walk heel to toe between them. I also practiced standing on one foot. I'd watch the second hand on the kitchen clock and stand like a stork for as long as I could, one foot shifting around on the floor. I would feel triumphant when I managed to finish half a minute without toppling over.

I hated working so hard at something I learned for the first time when I was two—equilibrium. But when the exacerbation ebbed, it left signs that it had been there. My balance had improved but wasn't normal. I was still unstable on my feet, still slightly wobbly, but I believed if I tried enough, it would all come back. It *had* to.

Anna's apartment was only three-fourths of a mile away, but I took a cab. I didn't know how far I could walk on my own now. I was afraid to find out.

I went when Anna was at work. I told myself she would exhibit a blend of superiority and pity I couldn't stomach. The truth was I knew I'd envy her strength and health. I'd envy them so much I couldn't bear it.

I usually stopped at Anna's (I considered it Anna's,

though I still paid half the rent) after my painting class. I painted a lot now. I was working on a painting of a nude woman. I thought I was painting a model, but now I see I was painting myself. The breasts and belly are mine; the long legs, the hair caught back in a ponytail.

The woman in the painting looks like she's falling on her head. The model was lying down, and I painted her with her head toward me and her body foreshortened. But if you didn't know that, you'd think she was falling upside down. Though her flesh is beautifully colored, her limbs are at peculiar angles—they aren't connected to her body correctly. She's falling apart.

I think that's only partly due to my lack of skill as a painter.

When the painting of the woman falling on her head was finished, I hung it on the wall at Anna's. I lay on the bed and looked at my things there. Books and more books, a typewriter, an easel, a lot of dust, a weight bench with a torn seat, its barbell, a pair of ballet slippers hanging on the wall (purely for aesthetics—I hadn't worn toe shoes for years), a squash racquet, a paddleball racquet, a racquetball racquet. Running shoes, riding boots. My rock-climbing harness hanging on the door.

While I was contamplating my things, Lex, a friend of Anna's, popped in.

Lex probably didn't like it when she saw me there. Confronting a person who is grieving is always difficult, but she sat down next to me and bravely tried to make conversation.

It wasn't long before MS (my only subject then) came up. Lex said simply and seriously, "If I knew how, I'd take the MS away." This was the nicest thing anyone had yet said. It acknowledged that a very bad thing had happened to me and also that she would stop it if she knew how. So far, other people had either pretended it wasn't so bad, or only talked about how bad it was for them.

For example, someone had said it would make me a better person. (Oh, great.) And someone had said that at least it had happened to me, I was a fighter. (Gee, thanks.) And someone had told me she'd spent a whole session talking to her shrink about it. (Do I care?) Before I'd started avoiding Anna she had told me it had taken an emotional toll on her.

"I'm so sorry it's taken an emotional toll on *you*," I had snapped.

"You're impossible," she replied.

I was. They were trying to be nice, but I felt I was being criticized for feeling so bad. I should be optimistic and have a good attitude and not feel sorry for myself. But I did feel sorry for myself, and envious of people in good health, as well as suspicious that they were glad I was out of the running. Now they wouldn't have to compete with me. (Now I think I was glad to have an excuse not to compete with them.) I was angry, self-absorbed, irascible, and very, very scared.

After giving me a hug, Lex left. The phone rang. It was the neurologist! Maybe he was calling to say he'd made a terrible mistake.

But the neurologist said, "I was wondering how you're doing emotionally."

"Okay," I said. "But sometimes I get so upset."

"That's appropriate," he said. So it's appropriate for me to be miserable, I thought. That means there wasn't a mistake. Dully, I asked about the spinal tap results.

"The CSF from the spinal tap showed a high value for oligoclonal bands, so there's been excessive myelin breakdown," the neurologist said. Myelin, the fatty sheath that surrounds the nerve, is what MS destroys. When the myelin, which acts something like insulation around a wire, is damaged, there is "static" in the central nervous system. Nerve messages get garbled, resulting in movement and sensory problems. Like mine.

So that is it: MS. Irrevocably.

All my tests were positive for multiple sclerosis—except the CAT scan. But most MS plaques, the scars or hardened places on the myelin that interfere with nerve conduction, don't show up on CAT. And all the other tests—the doctor's neurological exam and the evoked potentials and now the spinal tap—suggested MS. Though no test was conclusive by itself, together they made a pretty strong case. Which is the closest one can come to certainty with a diagnosis of MS. It must be that, because it isn't something else.

With many people, diagnosis is a trickier procedure than it was with me—there might be no sign of myelin breakdown in the CSF, for example. In fact, MS is often difficult to spot in its early stages. Symptoms often appear for only a few days or weeks and then disappear for months or even years, with the result that few people are diagnosed during their first attack. In fact, there is typically a lag of about three years between onset of symptoms and diagnosis.

Diagnosis can be aided, though, by a relatively new machine called an MRI, for magnetic resonance imaging. The visual image of the brain made by this machine shows up the plaques or scars of MS much more clearly than a CAT scan does.

An MRI is only able to make an image of the MS lesions, though; it can't do anything about them. I didn't have an MRI because it was expensive and for me seemed unnecessary. In 1984 an MRI test cost approximately $850–$950. It didn't seem worth it unless the diagnosis was more in doubt. Even the results of an MRI scan are not always conclusive.

The neurologist was still on the line. "I've made an appointment for you with Dr. Bornstein, the MS specialist we talked about," he said. On the day I was diagnosed, the neurologist had told me that trials for a new treatment for MS were being conducted at another New York City hospital. "The results so far look promising," he had said. "I'd like you to see the doctor conducting the trial."

If the substance Bornstein was testing—copolymer-1 or cop-1—turned out to be helpful to MS patients, I would have a head start by using it right after being diagnosed. It seemed that it was most effective on patients whose MS was still in an early stage. If I didn't take it during its trial period, it would be years before the stuff would be available, even if all went well. By then my disease might have progressed, and copolymer-1 would be less effective.

Of course, like so many other things that once looked promising in the treatment of MS, maybe copolymer-1 didn't really affect the disease at all. Nothing but time would tell.

The neurologist had said on the day of diagnosis, "If you do want to see Dr. Bornstein, I won't prescribe steroids for you. You are probably more likely to get into his trial if you haven't had any treatment for the disease."

I thought about it for a few minutes. "Okay."

Corticosteroids—prednisone or ACTH (adrenocorticotropic hormone)—are often prescribed for MS patients who are experiencing an exacerbation, an acute worsening of their symptoms. The steroids ameliorate the symptoms. It's thought that they work by reducing the swelling surrounding the damaged nerve fiber, but they don't seem to make a difference in the long-term course of the disease.

The appointment the neurologist had made with Dr. Bornstein was in three weeks. By then Dr. Bornstein would have received a letter with all the information about my "case." I thanked the neurologist and hung the phone up to brood. Well, I still had something to hope for. Maybe copolymer-1 would make everything all right again.

Anna (who really was a friend) called me at John's that night: there was a woman she wanted me to meet. Her name was Janet and she'd had MS for ten years. Anna thought she would be able to tell me what to expect.

The next day I waited outside a health food restaurant for Janet. Then I noticed a woman, heavyset, about my own age, walking toward me in a jerky manner. My heart sank; I knew this would be Janet. This jerkiness was not what I had hoped to see.

"Are you Moira?" the woman with the jerky gait said. "I'm sorry I'm late; I thought the restaurant was on a different block. Usually I'm better than this," she added with a deprecatory smile at her galumphing body. I felt guilty for bringing her out to comfort me, when my problems were so minor compared to hers. I felt bad because she seemed embarrassed about her incoordination. I also felt uneasy; I had wanted her to reassure me that MS would never do to me the things it was doing to her right now. She frightened me. I led the way indoors.

Janet's hand shook as she picked up her coffee cup with the decaf coffee. She had some books for me—one that John's father had already given me, called *The Swank Diet for Multiple Sclerosis*, as well as a British paperback that had a diet of its own to propose. And a book on acupuncture.

Then Janet dropped the first of several bombshells. She was blind in one eye. The disease had made her blind in both eyes at one point but that attack had ebbed, and vision had returned only to one eye. "Which eye?" I gasped.

"The right one."

"They both look fine."

"Yes." She smiled.

The blind eye moved as if it were sighted. After a first wash of sympathy I realized that this might happen to me. Irrationally, I began to hate her.

She told me about many strange things that I had never suspected were associated with MS—crazy mood swings, hysterical laughing, hideous depressions. Aphasia. I was morbidly fascinated. I thought she might be enjoying this a little: frightening me with the bizarre symptoms she had endured. Nevertheless, I was transfixed. Later, as I came to know more about the illness, I recalled the stories she had told me and doubted that they were all related to multiple sclerosis. Aphasia, for example, is extremely rare if it's *ever* caused by MS. But that day I believed her.

After lunch I walked a few blocks with her. Her gait was much smoother; she looked almost normal now.

Then I dashed away. I felt wild. There was nothing about her that was like me—*nothing*.

But after painting class one day I found out that we weren't so different. I decided to walk back to the loft. I crossed Washington Square and realized I was jerking like a puppet on a string. Was this real, or was I imagining it? People looked at me quickly, then looked away. Were they being polite, or had I become a ghost? Couldn't anyone see me anymore? I was afraid of myself. I thought if I waited it would get worse, so I tried to hurry. Walking by Grand Union, I stuck my fingers in the wire fence to hold myself up. I hurtled myself across Houston Street and leaned against the stone of John's building before going up. Inside, I stumbled to the bed and fell asleep.

I woke up a couple of hours later, and it was as if I had imagined it—I moved smoothly, like a normal person. I had never been jerky like that before. After I had fallen down during the exacerbation I had taken it very easy. Maybe I had been slightly uncoordinated at some point, but never so terribly. I didn't know yet that this was what I'd been left with—if I walked or ran too far, the damage to my nervous system became apparent. Most of the time I could pass for normal, but when I was hot or tired, I looked like I had cerebral palsy.

Characteristically, I made the situation melodramatic when I talked to myself. I thought: If this were the Middle Ages I would think I was possessed by the devil. Having MS *is* being possessed by the devil; this is how it feels to be possessed by the devil. Not yourself; gone, owned by someone else. Someone cruel.

When I remember those days, I remember amazement and fear.

When the day came to see Dr. Bornstein, John took off from work and borrowed the company car. Dr. Bornstein's hospital was Albert Einstein in the Bronx. It could have been on the moon (that's the way Manhattanites think). We got lost, of course, and drove around in frustrating circles while my tension mounted.

When we finally arrived, Dr. Bornstein was busy with another patient. After a short time, though, they were finished, and the patient stood beside her husband at the receptionist's desk, filling out insurance forms. She looked about forty, though she was leaning on a cane. She turned to speak to her husband and I noticed that it was hard for him to understand her, MS had impaired her speech so much. It seemed hard for her to get her mouth around the words.

Boy, I didn't want to be there.

Then Dr. Bornstein hailed me. He was a big man with a grizzled beard and a jovial manner. With a flowing robe instead of a white coat, he would have looked like an Old Testament prophet. He waved John into his office with me.

Though Dr. Bornstein was cheerful, I was spoiling for a fight. I wanted him to change the facts. They couldn't, mustn't be true.

I didn't say anything, but my restlessness must have shown. He looked over the information in my file—the test results and so on—and read the neurologist's letter out loud. Then he looked at me.

"You want a second opinion? I think you have MS."

So simply was I defeated.

"Of course, you're in remission," he said, staring at my stricken face. "Now tell me what you know about MS."

"It's terrible, terrible," I said, shaking my head. "It's terrible," I repeated.

"Not necessarily," he said, looking across the room as if someone stood there whom he was angry with. "It can be a terrible disease—I have patients who are bedbound and some who are dying. But I don't know why it's still described as an inexorable downward course. At least half my patients have mild cases."

Mild.

He described the individual course of MS as falling

somewhere on a bell curve, with some people having the disease so mildly that they are never even diagnosed and others having it so severely that they are bed-bound within months.

"Nearly fifty years ago, when I was a medical student doing autopsies, we found people whose neural tissue had the plaques that are definitive of multiple sclerosis. But they were perfectly healthy cadavers. They had had multiple sclerosis, but since they'd had no symptoms, they never knew it. You can have lots of scars and few symptoms, or few scars and lots of symptoms."

"How can that be!" I said.

"How can it be?" He shook his head.

4

Reading

Unfortunately, I did not fit the design for Dr. Bornstein's drug trial. People who had some history with MS were needed, so that some pattern or course of the disease was already established for them. Then Dr. Bornstein and his colleagues would be able to tell if cop-1 was making a difference in their disease progression. With someone so newly diagnosed, no one knew what to expect, so how could they tell if it was making a difference?

I was on my own.

But Dr. Bornstein said that "being on my own" wasn't necessarily so bad. The chances I'd have a mild case were better than I had thought. Not great, but better.

According to *Multiple Sclerosis: A Guide for Patients and Their Families* edited by Labe Scheinberg, M.D. ("Signs, Symptoms, and Course of the Disease" by Labe C. Scheinberg, New York: Raven Press, 1984, pp. 41–42) most people are between fifteen and fifty when MS first becomes symptomatic. More than 20 percent of people diagnosed with MS have a benign course. A sudden onset of symptoms is followed by one or two mild exacerbations that go into complete or nearly complete remission, in which all or most of the symptoms disappear. The few exacerbations take place during the early years, and then the disease appears to burn out—nothing more seems to happen. These people have a normal life-span (the average life expectancy of MS patients in general is thirty-five years after diagnosis). They develop little or no permanent disability, and most of the time no one would guess that they have MS.

Another 24 percent of patients follow the exacerbating-remitting course. Like the benign course, it begins suddenly, but the early attacks occur more frequently, and when the disease goes into remission, more symptoms remain behind. Still, the disease shows long periods of stability—months or even years. Some disability usually does develop, though.

The most common course is the chronic-relapsing course, affecting approximately 40 percent of patients. There are fewer and less complete remissions after exacerbations; eventually, there are no remissions. Disability increases slowly but steadily. About half the people in this category remain ambulatory; the other half use wheelchairs.

The most infamous form has an insidious onset but culminates in severe disability. Sometimes people deteriorate rapidly during the early years; sometimes they deteriorate slowly over several decades. Because there are no remissions, it is called the chronic-progressive course. About 15 percent of patients experience this most devastating form.

In the first years following diagnosis, though, the course that an individual's disease will take is anybody's guess, and some people change from one form of the disease to another. In other words, anything might happen. Nevertheless, most people with MS maintain the ability to walk, though some of them need aids—canes, crutches, or walkers.

•

No way to predict, and no way to control. MS is not a direct cause of craziness, but that there was no way to help myself was maddening, like sitting around waiting for the sword of Damocles to fall. Or maybe not to fall.

I remembered reading about "learned helplessness"—a psychologist's term for the passivity that animals develop when they are given shocks that are random and uncontrollable. Soon they stop trying to avoid the shocks. Even when it becomes possible for them to get away, they just lie there and take it. They've "learned" that nothing they can do makes any difference, so "Why bother?" seems to be their attitude.

"Learned helplessness" looks a lot like human depression. People who have MS are supposedly often depressed, but no one knows whether it's a direct result of the organic disorder—that it's related to the area in the brain where a certain scar has formed—or the indirect result of having an uncontrollable, unpredictable, and potentially terrible disease. Which is a good reason to get depressed. In any case, MS made me feel like a rat in a diabolical psychology experiment, with exacerbations as the unpredictable and unavoidable bolts from the blue.

I didn't want to learn that I was helpless, that there was nothing I could do. Though nothing is available (yet) to change the course of an individual's MS, I began to search for something to do.

I read everything I could get my hands on about MS. Though I would have laughed had anyone said I was looking for the cure (sort of like the quest for the Holy Grail), that idea must have been behind my new interest in medical textbooks and health food stores. A lot of the "information" was unnecessarily alarming—that people with MS would lose their wits and have to be carted around in less than ten years, for instance—but I had to open every book and pamphlet, no matter how outdated or how dubious the source.

I looked at many medical textbooks with photographs of demyelinated brain slices. "A sagittal section

with a Weigert stain shows areas of demyelination . . ."
The words would slide down the page and grow very
fat. The photographs would do the same; they'd slip off
and float in front of my face and pulse. But I had to look.
The elusive cure might reveal itself to me as I slogged
through *McAlpine's Multiple Sclerosis* or some other text a
mile or two above my very worried head. "Here I am —
THE CURE! Those laid-back scientists have overlooked
me, but I've been here all along!" Or perhaps some leaflet
off the rack in a health food store would deliver on its
promise of miracles.

Alas, this hasn't happened yet.

I also went to a homeopath. But I think you have to
have faith in those pills for them to work. I didn't, and
they didn't. But I won't pooh-pooh something I don't
understand. Maybe I'll try homeopathy again someday.

I stayed with John until the spring. I don't think he
was too thrilled that I had entrenched myself in his life
again. The most solid of relationships are strained by
something like multiple sclerosis—and we had broken
up already and were supposed to be "just friends." John
had no responsibility for me, but I was acting as if he did.

I also blush to admit that I may have used the MS
as emotional blackmail. How could he be so heartless as
to throw me out now—weak, vulnerable me? And many
people think stress triggers exacerbations (whether it
really does isn't clear yet). How could he live with himself
if he caused me to experience stress and I had an exacerbation? What was he, a brute?

Well, he wasn't, and this ruse worked for about four
months. Actually, I don't know how much of that
thought process is real—it certainly wasn't conscious. I
would have gagged if I thought I was doing that. But as
I've been told, the best-kept secrets are the ones we keep
from ourselves.

In any case, I ended up moving out again—inevit-
ably, I guess. I went back to the house where I grew up.
I think this was a bad move; it made me feel dependent
and defeated. Twenty-nine years old, and she can't live

alone on her own in the city, an incipient cripple. This disparaging word was a description I wouldn't use for someone else, but it suited the way I thought about myself then. When I read Nancy Maire's excellent book, *Plaintext*, and saw how she used "crippled" to describe what MS had done to her, I decided to use it, too.

Thank God (or thank John), I didn't stay in Connecticut even for the summer.

Before I left New York, I had my first piece of good luck—I talked to Holly.

I'd known Holly for years. She was often at the parties at John's loft. But all I knew about her was that she was blonde and attractive and a painter. We had a lot of friends in common.

One day I ran into her former boyfriend, another painter, named Carlos. He asked me how I was. I took this as my cue to burst into tears, but I did manage to tell him that I'd found out that I had MS. I expected him to be properly appalled, so I was stunned at his matter-of-fact reply.

"Call Holly. She's had MS for years—she knows what it's like."

"Holly!"

I didn't call her right away; I kept losing her number. I felt shy. I had talked about MS to just about anybody who would listen—unknown women in the locker room, the instructor of my nonaerobic exercise class—but I still felt alone and singled out by it. But Holly would understand completely. Suddenly I felt exposed. What was I afraid she was going to see?

I was pretty sure of what she *wouldn't* see—the courageous person that other people thought they saw (or said they did). Holly would know just how scared and hurt I was. She wouldn't be impressed by my bravado, my claims that I'd lick this thing and still run a marathon or compete in a triathlon. The bluster was to hide my fragility, the thought that maybe I can't.

Holly wouldn't be fooled by my bluster. She'd know exactly what the calamitous possibilities were. She'd also

know that they didn't happen to everyone. Nor would
she pretend to think I was engaged in a noble struggle—
living with something I didn't choose and couldn't
change. There is nothing noble about that.

At last I phoned her; she was expecting me.

Holly had been diagnosed six years earlier. I was
envious. The neurologist had said that it took about five
years to tell whether a person's disease was benign or
not (although I've heard differing opinions since). But if
he was right, Holly's course was benign. Did she walk
smoothly now? She did. Lose her balance a little? Nope.

Would I be like Holly, or would MS cripple me? She
said that I reminded her of how she had been right after
being diagnosed: scared, sure that every little thing had
some dire meaning. "See a shrink," she said. "It helps."
She'd seen an analyst since being diagnosed. I thought,
Why not? Any port in a storm.

Before following her suggestion, though, I moved
back home. Everything seemed so green in Connecticut,
especially after the gray of New York. Green is the color
of hope, I told myself; of new beginnings. I was starting
over. Where better to start over than at home?

I filled my old room with boxes of books: the eigh-
teenth-century literature phase, the I-think-I'll-be-a-law-
yer phase, the feminist phase. I set up my typewriter,
stacked my paintings in green plastic garbage bags (which
probably improved them), stuffed the closet with business clothes, woolen suits and silk blouses. It had been
a long time since I'd worn that sort of thing. Now I
dressed like a teenage boy: sneakers, jeans, sweatshirts.

My self-important and unsentimental cat roamed up
and down the stairs while I installed a pull-up bar in my
bedroom doorway, set up my 10-speed on rollers in the
garage, put my weight bench and dumbbells in the musty
cellar, and lay on my old bed surveying my new-old
abode.

I remember that summer as if it happened under
water. The sounds I recall seem muffled and everything
I saw looked slightly distorted.

There wasn't much to do. I'd wake up late, and very slowly. Then I'd lie in bed for who knows how long. Finally I'd realize I was hungry or had to go to the bathroom, so I'd drag myself up, feed the frantic cat, turn the radio on, and sit in the kitchen. There'd be nobody else in the house—my parents lived across town with my grandmother now. So I turned the radio up even louder and drank a cup of tea. Half an hour later I'd be ready for the Cheerios. Before you knew it, it was noon.

But I wasn't depressed. I wasn't depressed at all! Though I moved through the morning as if swimming through quicksand, I told myself I wasn't depressed; just slow in getting started.

What I did next I used to think was proof of my strong state of mind. I went running.

My idea was to take the same route I took during high school when I went running with my dog. Leaping over hedges, scampering up hills (or so I fondly "remembered"). But within five minutes I found out some modifications had to be made. I no longer scampered; I plodded.

Many, though not all, people with MS find that heat makes their symptoms worse. This seems to be the case with me. So it was stupid and cruel to myself to run during the middle of the day. It was so hot and muggy then that any sensible person would choose another time for running. I guess I wanted to run when it was hardest.

I climbed the hill to its flat top and took off.

The first quarter mile felt great. Sun glinted off the cars by the side of the road and off the mica specks under my feet. At the end of the street was a big old willow; that was the quarter-mile mark. After passing it, I turned around and jogged back to the stop sign where I'd started. When I was almost there, I noticed that I had slowed down a lot and that the toe of my left foot nicked the ground, once, twice.

This made me furious. "Up," I said to my left foot, "up." At last I was at the stop sign. That's all I did the first two weeks: a humble half mile. The next week I got

back to the stop sign and took a right. This was the dead
end with the hedges I remembered leaping over. Now
when I got to the hedges, I sat down.

By then I was only hopping up and down anyhow.
If I was going forward at all, it wasn't much. I had pushed
myself only three-fourths of a mile, and the last quarter
mile made me weak and trembly, with a spastic right leg.

Amazing that such a short time before I wouldn't
even have started counting at half a mile. I would hardly
have noticed it.

I flopped down on the grass and watched the dogs
that lived across the street come halfway out into the
road to howl at me. I howled back; I felt that mean.

Did I romanticize the situation (which I privately
called "my plight")? You bet. While I flopped on the grass
I invented a fantasy.

By "running," I was fighting back against an intol-
erable situation, I said to myself. I was making the most
of what strength I had, and nobly refusing to accept the
"slings and arrows of outrageous fortune." I thought
there was something heroic—sad but valiant—about
my run.

But the stumbling at the end. The exhaustion. It
wasn't fair.

There I sat, brooding by the side of the road. In some
ways I was a fairly immature twenty-nine-year-old, and,
face it, this was a pretty trying time. I was being forced
to change, and I didn't want to. I didn't want to let athletic
Moira go. Especially when I didn't know who would
replace her.

When my strength came back, I walked slowly home.

On other days, I swam a mile at the Y or rode my bike
in the garage or lifted weights in the cellar with the radio
on loud. In the afternoons I went to the library to work
on my thesis and comb the card catalog for books on MS.
In the evening I collapsed into bed moaning about how
the disease made me tired.

I got around either by taking the occasional bus or

by having my parents drive me. This made me feel shamefully dependent, but that's the way it was.

I didn't drive. I had a license, which I got when I was sixteen, but I hadn't been behind the steering wheel for years. In the city, no one needed a car; out of the city, John drove; at home, my sisters drove. But now I felt marooned.

Suppose I wanted to do something respectable, like go to the library: I had to call my mother. Suppose I wanted to do something not-so-respectable (well, I might)—like shop for a garter belt. Then forget it.

Just more evidence of how dependent I was for a twenty-nine-year-old (and must have wanted to be). Because it didn't have to be that way.

True, it's just as well that after seven years in the passenger's seat, I didn't lean over, turn the key in the ignition, and zoom off. That would have been really self-destructive. But I could have kept in driving practice throughout those years—after all, my sisters did.

Not driving was okay, I told myself then, because, in and of itself, it's not all that important. This would have been true; but for me, not driving was a way of being taken care of. (A few years later, I took some brush-up lessons and my license meant something again.) I thought I would relearn to drive that summer. But—and maybe I shouldn't have been surprised—the proposition met with disapproval. Just because I wanted to change, why should everybody around me change, too? If I started to drive myself around again, my parents wouldn't have even one baby left—the other girls had apparently grown up. There was only me to continue the job of being the baby, and I was pretty good at it.

My mother had read a story by Berton Roueché in the *New Yorker* about a young woman with a different autoimmune disease—myasthenia gravis, a neuromuscular condition about which I know very little. No matter that the diseases were different—they were enough alike to my mother to support her stance in not letting me drive. The woman with myasthenia gravis in the story was so weak at one point that she couldn't depress the brake when she was in an intersection. This was proof positive that I, who had a different disease, shouldn't relearn to drive.

But that didn't keep me at home. It just meant she or my father had to drive me to crazy places. I joined a painting group about forty minutes away. Twice a week one or the other drove me to the painting group early in the morning. With paints and outdoor easels, the painting group members (mostly elderly ladies with lots of money) braved the wilds of Connecticut to draw babbling brooks with curving bridges and groups of bored-looking cows. Most of them preferred painting pictures of barns.

I could stand at my easel for hours without my legs aching—I guess they didn't complain because they weren't the focus of my attention. This made me confident enough so that a few times I stopped off at a stable on the way home and tried riding again—a lumpy old mare named Potatoes. But an hour in the sun on her, just walking and trotting, made me very wobbly. I would have been better painting Potatoes than riding her—and that's not saying much. In any case, I wasn't ready to admit it.

Things went along in this fashion for a couple of months. Then one night it happened: the *second exacerbation.*

I was lying in bed waiting to fall asleep when my left hand started tingling. An odd sort of tingling, not quite like anything I'd felt before. I sat bolt upright and shook my hand. I rubbed it. It still tingled.

Tingling is a symptom of MS—one of its mildest symptoms. It's annoying and frightening, but it doesn't prevent you from doing anything.

"Ah, but suppose it's the harbinger of something much worse?" I said to myself.

"Ah, but suppose it isn't?" my rational self said back.

Ignoring that remark, I rubbed my hand and raved: "Two exacerbations within a few months! This must be a sign that things will get much worse."

"Maybe not," my rational self said, now truly exasperated. "Maybe not."

I was really scared. But it's also true that I was getting off on my alarm and doing a good job of escalating it into terror. In any case, I didn't want to be alone with either the fear or the thrill. So I called Cynthia in the middle of the night.

She answered the phone and listened to my story. Then she brought out an arsenal of reasons why the tingling wasn't what I thought.

"Tingling? But that happens to me all the time! Maybe you were lying on your hand. Shake it around."

"I tried that."

"Oh. Well, rub it, then."

I wasn't getting very far. I said, "All right, well, good night."

I sat on the floor and promised the God I still said I didn't believe in that I'd stop doing it—whatever it was—if only he'd let me get better. Please, God.

The next day the tingling started in the other hand. I had few distractions at home, so I was able to concentrate on it. During the next few weeks I fanned the flames of the anxiety it caused and in no time my preoccupation was a full-blown obsession. I noted how the tingling moved from one hand to the other, then into my feet, then back into my hands.

I telephoned my internist. He said, not unsympathetically, "Wait it out." Eventually the tingling would subside on its own. Any drug he could prescribe had side effects that were worse than tingling.

But fortitude was in short supply where I lived.

I telephoned my neurologist. He sounded concerned but told me to call back if something worse happened.

I telephoned my specialist. "Tingling? That's all?" He had patients who were sick.

Finally I telephoned Holly. "Tingling is the lowest rung on the ladder," she said.

"But it's never happened to me before."

"Well, it's happened to me. Just don't think about it," she said firmly.

"I can't help it," I said miserably.

"Yes you can. It's probably the hardest thing you've ever had to do," she said more gently. "Forget it."

On the third day of the tingling, having exhausted my phone book, I decided it was up to me to do something. I started off by taking inventory.

Yes, I could still move all the parts: I wiggled my fingers, I wiggled my toes. I tested my proprioception—my sense of where I was in space. I closed my eyes and touched the index finger of my right hand to my nose, then the index finger of my left hand. Then both index fingers together in front of me.

The first time I tried this, the fingers didn't quite meet and I had to peek; the second time I got them to touch with my eyes closed. So then I ran the heel of my left foot down my right shin. Speedy and smooth. When I tried to do the same with my right heel and left shin, it wasn't so straight or so smooth—there was an awkward moment when it wobbled—but it wasn't too bad, anyway no different from usual. (I'd done this before.) I stood on one foot and watched the clock for half a minute, then on the other foot. No noticeable difference.

So I lifted weights. No difference. I tried the bike. The same. Only my thoughts seemed affected by the tingling—and they were getting pretty skewed. I couldn't think about anything else; it was excruciatingly boring, but it seemed I couldn't help it.

I'd read stories in magazines about people who used a technique called "imaging" to rally their immune systems. They imagined their immune systems overcoming foreign invaders. Supposedly, their immune systems were enhanced by this technique and defended their bodies with greater success. Whether or not any benefit had been proven, imaging seemed worth trying; even if it was a straw, as far as I knew, there were no logs floating around.

Of course there was a glitch. In all the stories I had read, there was an outside invader—a bacteria or virus. Patients imagined this invader as an evil army that their good army—the cells of their own immune systems—fought and ultimately vanquished.

But MS is commonly thought to be an autoimmune disease in which the immune system turns on the body it is supposed to be protecting. Although something from the outside—a virus, say—may indeed trigger the autoimmune response, it seems to be the immune system itself that actually wreaks the havoc and destroys the myelin surrounding the nerve fibers.

For me, this was a sticking point. It would be awful if my immune system won the war. That would mean it had vanquished my myelin. I needed my myelin. And I needed my immune system, too.

I decided that my immune system just didn't recognize my myelin as its own. It thought the oligodendroglial cells (great word, oligondendroglia) that made up the myelin were foreign troops and attacked them. I figured if I could get the immune system to recognize the oligodendroglia (hey, guys, it's me—Ollie), it would call off the war.

The cell in the immune system that gives the all-clear to the disease-fighting cells is called the suppressor T cell. During an exacerbation, the suppressor T cells seem to disappear, though they do not totally. They return when the disease goes into remission. I figured that meant the disease-fighting cells chewed up the myelin only while the suppressor T cells were away; when they came back, they called the battle—or exacerbation—off.

This is no explanation, of course, for what really

happens in MS. Alas, it's much more complicated. In fact, no one understands it yet. But this is the way I thought about it then.

I sat cross-legged on my bed and began deep breathing. I thought back to the stable where I used to work and where the MS began. Doberman pinschers met me at the stable's half-door and began to snarl. They were the disease-fighting cells of the immune system and were out to get me (representing the myelin), whom they didn't recognize. They thought I was an invading virus they should destroy fast. They barked and snarled and let me know they meant business.

When, lo and behold, the watchman cometh. Playing the part of a suppressor T cell, he sat down on the mounting block. "Lie down," he said to the dogs. "Lie down."

They did. Not all at once, but slowly and reluctantly, whimpering and looking confused. The watchman patted a dog on the head. "All the dogs lie down," he said.

It wasn't really the dogs' fault for attacking the myelin; they mistook it for something else. They were trying to protect my body.

I used the fantasy several times a day. I'd like to say this is how I cured my MS, or at least how I stopped the tingling. But what the fantasy did was this: It reduced the tingling or else it just distracted me so that I didn't notice it as much. Who knows which? But I felt better.

A few weeks later I went to Regina's wedding, still tingling on and off. I probably walked around looking woeful though I should have been happy—my new brother-in-law seemed great, and my sister looked radiant. The day was sunny and there were lots of flowers in the church.

Tingling through the wedding kept Poor Me at the center of my thoughts—I mean, that was understandable, wasn't it? so who could blame me—instead of my radiantly happy younger sister. It distracted me from the envy that might otherwise have clobbered me over the head.

Ah, the uses of illness—how did I ever do without them?

John was at the wedding. I hadn't quite given up on trying to impress him with the sadness of my lot, so I told him a few times with great soberness that I was tingling. I was scared and afraid no one, except possibly John, could ever love me. Maybe he would for old times' sake. Anyway, despite these barely disguised pleas (take care of me!) it was good to be with him again, laughing and easy, and I think vice versa.

A few weeks later he called me from New York. "You'll find something different next time you see me," he said mysteriously. A few minutes after we hung up I thought I knew. He had gone rock climbing with some friends of ours over the weekend. I called back.

"It's your arm," I said. "You broke it."

But it was his leg. He didn't know how bad it was yet, but it seemed twice its normal size. He'd fallen on a ledge while leading a climb. His leg wasn't broken but something bad had happened to it. He'd know more that afternoon after he saw a doctor. It hurt.

That afternoon he was told he had torn some ligaments and damaged some cartilage. He was scheduled for an operation. I got on the train. I had to take care of him!

When I got to the city, I went to his loft, watered the plants, fed the cats. Then I went to the hospital where John was sitting in a nightshirt surrounded by legal pads, the lawyer hard at work.

John was terribly interested in what they were going to do to his leg. He drew lots of knees on the yellow pads, with all their inner connections so I could picture what was to happen. I was polite. I pretended to be entranced even when he showed me for the third time. He was clearly in pain—in the middle of a conversation he'd stop and roll his eyes up in a peculiar and frightening way. After they operated on his knee, he would be in even greater pain for a while. "But I'm lucky," he told me. "I'm going to have microsurgery. Only years ago a fall like that would have left me with a permanent limp."

It was left hanging in the air that I was the one with the permanent (though occasional) limp.

John was operated on. I stayed at the loft, taking care of the four cats and two parrots, and visited him every day at the hospital.

He hurt. Because the hospital staff was on strike, he missed his pain-killing drugs several times. I was put on alert; I set my alarm and called him in the middle of the night to see if they'd remembered his narcotic. If not, he called someone then, before the last dose's effect wore off.

After five days, he came home. The leg that had been operated on had staples in it. It had become skinny and strange-looking next to the other muscular limb; I called it his Biafran leg. He was using crutches; eventually he had a cane.

Some of my feelings weren't very nice. Although I felt bad for John, I was glad that I was the able-bodied one. He didn't run ahead of me now; I had to wait up for him. Unkind feelings seeped out: Now he'd know how it felt. But I still wanted him to get better. I just wanted to get better, too. Gradually he did get better, and I started looking for a new place to stay.

5

Meeting Sam

My friend Patrick was going to Nicaragua to help the Sandinistas build bridges. His two cats needed company for the time he'd be gone, and he needed someone to pay a few months' rent. I moved out of John's loft again.

It was early in the fall when I moved into Patrick's studio on the Upper West Side. He had two fat cats. I brought one scrawny, hyper one. My only chore was to feed them; that was all I had to do.

I cried uncontrollably at the most inoffensive things. Once it was a movie in which a fire was set in someone's loft. There were lots of big paintings that burned and the girl's father died in the fire. At the movie I cried and cried—embarrassing hiccoughing sobs I could not squelch.

I dreamed of a figure floating facedown in a river. It didn't have to get up again.

I went to the gym a lot. Lots of depressed people hang out at the gym; it's something to do and someplace to be. I pushed around weights in the same old weight room, did three sets of biceps curls, three sets of kickbacks, just as if everything were the same. As if biceps curls mattered. As if there was anything left that mattered. Still, I dawdled in the locker room, getting dressed slowly, so I didn't have to leave. I brightly said hello to people I knew only vaguely and milled about with NYU students, pretending things hadn't irrevocably and horribly changed.

One day I was hanging out in the weight room waiting for a leg machine, when a voice said something to me about it being so hot. I turned around.

He was about my height and had black wavy hair. He said he was so hot.

Yeah.

Then he asked me what my age was. Probably not right away, probably after saying something friendly and inconsequential that I can't remember now. "How old are you?" he said. I remember that.

Well, clearly, I wasn't an undergraduate. (Well, clearly, neither was he.) "Twenty-nine," I said, which I would be for almost another week.

I asked him what he did. He said he was a neuroscientist. Neuroscience! "I'm very interested in that," I said. "For, uh, personal reasons." Then I demurely looked away.

I wish I hadn't done that. Three years later, I still wish I hadn't done that.

"What neurological disease do you have?" he said.

I thought for a very short moment of saying it wasn't me, it was my mother or my sister, but this didn't seem fair. Anyway, for all sorts of reasons, I didn't lie.

"MS," I said. I know I shouldn't be ashamed of it any more than I should be proud of it. But I was a little ashamed, and still am, at times.

But the hot neuroscientist didn't looked horrified. He just looked at me. He seemed receptive. "It doesn't affect your strength," he said, pointing toward the weight machines. "It just makes you fatigued?" I started to talk.

MS didn't make me weak, it didn't even make me fatigued! (Actually, it makes me weak only when it makes me fatigued. But I get fatigued quickly when I do anything aerobic or repetitious—like walking or running or just cleaning the house.) I told him about copolymer-1 (pretending to know just what "polypeptide" means) and how I couldn't get into the cop-1 trial and did he think that was so bad? Without waiting for an answer I told him about the letter I'd received from someone who headed an MS research team (I'd sent letters to anyplace where a research project was under way). And then another letter some scientists sent me about remyelination in animals. (The neuroscientists who answered my letters were very kind. They must get a lot of letters, and they really don't have the answers yet.) The neuroscientist I was talking to mashed up rat brains and looked for neurochemical changes in the rats who just had learned mazes. He listened politely.

Then he said, "I know a woman who had one attack and hasn't had another for ten years."

So I told him about Holly. I said, "She's so beautiful, I thought, 'She can't have MS!' " (I wanted him to think the same about me.) I was shifting back and forth from one foot to the other, so I leaned against one of the weight machines. I was afraid he would notice how I stood with my feet wide apart to keep my balance. I was afraid he would name it: Aha! The typical compensatory wide-based stance adopted by people who are ataxic. Ataxic: off-balance. I was splay-legged like a brand-new foal. And as trembly as one. (I don't think the trembling had anything to do with MS, though.)

Finally I said, "This is making me nervous. I want to stop." We said good-bye and separated.

I started to feel bad. I didn't even know him, but I'd subjected him to a grueling half hour of listening. I found him and apologized.

———————

I went "home" to Patrick's studio. The apology wasn't enough, so I wrote a letter. I wrote it and reread it and wrote it again. I didn't know his address, I didn't even know his last name! I knew where he worked, though. I'd send the letter there.

If only I knew his name!

I never did send the letter, but I saw him at the gym about two weeks later. He wasn't really *that* good-looking. He walked over to me and asked what I had done for Halloween. There was an easy answer (nothing), but instead of saying that I turned on my heel and went over to a weight machine to do something for my still-there muscles. He wandered off, not looking perturbed, though I was sure he was.

Now I had two reasons for remorse! I had been a medical bore and I had snubbed him at the gym.

I started going to the gym even more frequently. I accidentally bumped into the neuroscientist again. This time instead of going on and on about MS, I went on and on about my journalism thesis on diplomatic immunity, which had been edited and was going to be published in a law magazine. I thought he'd be impressed.

He looked annoyed.

Then I asked him to hold my shoulders down while I did pull-downs. I needed him for all three sets. Then I started touching him when we talked. Just little taps on the arm to emphasize important phrases. At last, he asked me for my phone number.

I had nothing to write it on. "Will you remember it if I just say it?"

"Of course, I'm a memory expert," he said modestly. So I told him.

Thus began the saga of Sam. I have an urge to say here that he called that night, a cure was found for MS, I beat him to the Nobel Prize, and despite that we rode into the sunset and lived happily ever after.

Three weeks passed and we bumped into each other at the gym again. "I lost the paper with your number," he explained. I nodded understandingly.

That should have been enough. I should have

sniffed, turned on my heel, and said, "His loss." (It *would* have been.)

Instead I persisted in being aggressively available. (I'm embarrassed by this now; I wish it were longer ago.) I sent him mystifying letters. I made phone calls to ask him out.

He was always polite, but he was always busy.

Part of me says, Come on, Griffin, having a crush on someone is not exactly out of the ordinary. And he wasn't totally unsusceptible. We did go out a few times, eventually.

But only a few.

Why didn't Sam find me irresistible? I couldn't fathom it. I told myself that I wasn't really intellectually pretentious, even if I had laid on the stuff about diplomatic immunity a little thick. And what if I had a neurological disease and he was a neuroscientist? That just meant he'd know that a person could have MS for a long time (even an entire lifetime) and not get worse. So he wouldn't worry. It wasn't as if I were hoping he could do something for me.

I used to say, "Knowledge is power"—maybe I *did* think he could do something for me. I don't think that was a big part of my crush on him, though it must have played some role. His area of neuroscience was so far afield from anything that might help me, and I understood that. However, I make no claims to rationality here.

We continued to see each other at the gym. I really did enjoy talking to him and even listening—though I did a lot less of that. Sam might have been a friend of mine, but friendship wasn't understood by me then. I had male "friends," but only ones I thought, or hoped, were in some sort of sexual thralldom. Or who thought the MS was "poignant," or so they said, while I was plain afraid of it. I thought it was ugly; I thought it was repulsive.

I have no idea what Sam thought. He was pretty good at keeping his thoughts to himself. In any case, I wasn't a "poor woman." I was scheming and conniving. But I was out of luck with Sam.

Winter arrived, and Patrick returned. I rented an apartment with a couple of roommates and got a job through *The New York Times* working on another directory. I didn't give up being infatuated with Sam anywhere near soon enough. I still think it wouldn't have hurt him to be more cooperative, but still it was fun to have a crush and, at least in the beginning, good for me. Instead of lying on my bed staring at the ceiling until noon, I got up. Life isn't over, I realized; in fact, it's just begun. I wanted to look good again; I wanted a job; I wanted to write.

And after work, I went to Achilles. Achilles was a division of the New York Road Runners Club, set up especially for disabled people who wanted to "run." I had almost stopped running that year because when you fall in New York, lots of people see you. I fell frequently, or at least got spastic and jerky when I ran. I was normal when I started, but after that first half mile, I couldn't take it.

I thought I had to keep running, though—without it, I would get weak. Besides, giving it up would be a defeat. I told myself I had to do it. Perhaps if I joined Achilles, I would run regularly again. Why would I be embarrassed when my feet started to flap if I was with other people whose bodies had problems? I read about Achilles in the paper on Sunday, and called the NYRR Club on Monday.

A woman answered. She said she was a social worker who was also a runner, and once a week she took some of the Achilles members around Central Park. I guessed she took me for a journalist from the way she answered my questions. Reluctantly I blurted out that I wanted to be one of the Achilles runners, and her whole aspect changed—which is what I had hoped and feared. She was very nice to me but I decided that she gushed. (Now, I doubt that was true. Besides, no matter how she had acted, I would have found it insulting. I was so defensive in those days, I couldn't admit that anyone could treat me right.) Nevertheless, she told me to come on Wednesday evening, and I did.

It was dark Wednesday evening, and cold. I stood outside the beautiful old building where the NYRR Club was housed and wondered if I should go in. I wasn't a runner anymore, I said to myself; I was a disabled runner, something different. I hated myself for that. I went in.

The Achilles Club met in the library, said some people selling NYRR Club T-shirts. I hoped they couldn't tell why I asked.

During the next few months I "ran" with the Achilles club. I put quotation marks around "ran," because it wasn't normal running. It could just as easily have been called rowing—it bore so little resemblance to the usual sort of running. Everyone in Achilles had a different style. There were a few people who "ran" in wheelchairs. There was a woman with cerebral palsy who swung through her crutches (she went a lot faster and farther than I could go, I might add). There was a Scottish man who had had a stroke. There were a couple of blind runners. They ran tied to their sighted partners. And there was the president of the club, who only had one leg and wore a prosthesis. He skipped when he ran.

But Achilles was not for me—at least not then. I hope I seemed nonchalant as I stumbled around the Delacorte Oval in Central Park for the second time, but I was screaming inside. I couldn't believe I had come to that.

Besides identifying me as disabled, Achilles was hard for me because it reminded me of camp: the organized activities, the earnest counselors, the buddy system. "And who are you with today, Moira?" the Achilles volunteer asked, and I said, "I'm with . . . Joe!"

"But he didn't come today. Who did you say you're running with?"

"I'm with Marilyn, then," I said, smiling at Marilyn, who grinned at me from her wheelchair.

I suppose it was a good idea for us to go "running" in small groups. It was practical as well as friendly. Who knows, maybe the NYRR Club would be sued by the irate family of an Achilles member if he or she got hurt while trudging around the runners' paths of the park alone on a meeting night. I suppose a solitary disabled runner would be tantalizing to New York's muggers. The buddy system (which I don't think was ever called that) still felt regressive to me, but I had such a big chip on my shoulder that I doubt anything would have felt right.

One of our organized activities was stretching in the park. During the winter we did our stretching in the library, but once it was spring, we went *en masse* to Central Park and stretched outdoors.

We made a circle. Usually there were between twelve and twenty of us, some accompanied by crutches, canes, or wheelchairs. Some of the people running by with their muscular legs in sexy skintight latex stopped short and watched us. Then the volunteers' voices grew odd and self-conscious as they led the stretching exercises. "Reach up, *up!* as high as you can go . . . Now reach down, down, *down* as low as you can go." Everyone did what he could.

"I feel like I'm on *Romper Room*," I said to another Achilles member as I held on to somebody's wheelchair and bent this way and that. I held on to the wheelchair because although my stretching was good, my balance was awful. We snickered. It's hard to be nice or "have a good attitude" when you feel that you're a spectacle.

One of the best things Achilles did for me, though, was to introduce me to a lot of people with different disabilities. The abnormal was normal there, and became unimportant. It made me feel less sorry for myself, less special and singled out for disaster. Living with MS—at least with my degree of involvement—is not pleasant, but it's not such a big deal compared to other disabilities.

The first time I really knew I wasn't especially blighted was about nine months into it when I met the other people at Achilles.

There's a big danger of becoming too involved with disability by participating in something like Achilles, though, especially for someone whose problems really don't have to be a big part of his or her life. It's easy to develop an attitude of us, the disabled, versus them, people who are apparently normal. But most people have problems, although they aren't always visible or physical. Disabled people do not have a monopoly on trouble.

It might be a commonplace to most people, but for me it was news that disabled people are full-fledged individuals with hopes and hates and loves. I probably paid lip service to that thought for years, but I didn't really believe it.

Until I joined Achilles, I saw disabled people simply as "The Disabled" and thought disability was the main, if not the only, fact of their lives.

For a long time disability was the main fact of my life. Not at all in actuality, but in the way I thought about myself. Disability was my important, clandestine life, and Achilles was the main part of that life. Away from Achilles I could "pass" for normal. If I rode my stationary bike and that made me tired and spastic, I could lie down on my bed and nobody had to know. But "running" in Central Park made my disability blatant. The whole question of secrecy and disclosure is still a big one for me. The disabled life was often cruel, but in its own way, it was seductive.

Right here I have to ask myself: Am I a Disabled Person? Disabled for what? I need to know. I'm disabled for hiking and for rock climbing, certainly, and I'm not going to take another bicycle trip around Vermont like I did in my early twenties unless something truly unexpected happens. But I'm not disabled for writing or painting or getting a quart of milk at the grocery store or walking to the subway or even taking a nonaerobic exercise class. I guess everybody needs to ask that question: disabled for what?

At first I ran because "I can't believe this" and "I'm no quitter—I'm going to beat this." But after a while I ran, oddly enough, because I'm lazy. Life is too hard, I thought, and still sometimes think; maybe people will expect less of me if I'm crippled. That's what beggars in the subway seem to think: that people will think it impossible for them to be responsible, real people, because they have a disability. I hate to remember this period in my life because I believe that I was like a beggar in the subway. I think part of the reason I went to Achilles was because there I felt disabled. (I never was aware of thinking this way then, believe me.) But this notion—that I can get by with less, that I *ought* to get by with less—is a terribly hard one to give up.

I also ran to punish myself for getting MS. Flailing about as I did when the symptoms developed was the most emotionally excruciating thing I could do, and I did it over and over.

Roger Hartnett, an Achilles member, had ideas about MS, too. I was the first person with MS who joined Achilles, though others did later. Maybe he understands the disease better now. I wondered if he was right, but I wasn't willing to test his idea out. He thought that if the appearance of symptoms came on with a rise in body temperature caused by aerobic exercise, I should just keep on going—the body temperature would level off eventually, he thought, and so would my symptoms.

But early exhaustion was one of my symptoms, and when I got hot enough, I couldn't keep my balance even with a cane. I was angry already, and I thought this idea was unrealistic, even impossible, so I felt angrier. On the other hand, the exercise was definitely good for me—but the emotional pain outweighed the physical benefits.

I ran around the Delacorte Oval, but others went the three miles around the park. Disability meant something different to everyone. Some of the people finished marathon after marathon and were strong and fit, but never looked normal. They always walked with a severe limp or were spastic or needed crutches, while I could pass for normal most of the time but couldn't run a mile.

The first time I ever felt comfortable enough to laugh at my symptoms was at Achilles. I was on the way to the oval with Mike, who was tall and thin and walked a little lopsided because he had cerebral palsy, and Marilyn, in her wheelchair. I sat down on a guard rail for a moment. Before I knew what was happening, I toppled over backward and was on the ground with my feet in the air. I laughed and laughed. With most people, I would have been so embarrassed. "Be careful!" Marilyn scolded me as she rolled up. "Stay on the inside of my chair. Keep away from those cars!"

So I did.

Delacorte Castle was lighted up in the dark, and you could see the bright city rimming the park. Everything looked mysterious. I ran and then I walked, and then I changed into someone who could hardly walk.

I was at Achilles when I heard Mike say he'd rather be lifting weights.

"Me, too!" I said. "I lift all the time."

Mike enjoys being a confidant. Since I like to talk and philosophize, we became friends, and one day I went to his gym.

Mike started lifting weights when he was fourteen, thirty years ago. The last time I asked, he was bench-pressing 285 pounds. He seemed to think I should, too. He's a slave driver. Lots of women threw themselves at Mike, just for a hug and a squeeze, nothing more. And Mike was happy to oblige. Mike was married to a woman who also had CP. I wondered—didn't the women who threw themselves at Mike realize that he was a man like any other? Sometimes I suspected he was playing "the innocent cripple" just to get another squeeze.

I accompanied Mike to his gym several times, but

we really had different workouts, so I went back to my own gym for lifting.

I was still going to Achilles and to my dull job, when I decided to write an article. Having MS was still so bewildering to me; maybe it always will be. But I thought if I wrote it all down I would get it straight; I would teach myself how to think about it.

No writing assignment ever gripped me like that article did. I worked on it until late at night and got up early to work on it again. The article grew so long most magazines wouldn't publish it, so I pared it down.

In two or three weeks I mailed it to the psychology director at a major women's magazine with a health and independence slant. I thought the piece was just right for them, even if they didn't generally publish stories of that kind. Maybe they'd publish mine.

While I was waiting to hear from them, I got laid off because of budget cuts. After telling me that I'd have to go, my boss said, "Why don't you try writing a book?"

I told him about the article. He said he'd like to read it, and I just happened to have a copy on me. He read it, said he liked it, and we outlined *The Question and Answer Book on MS* together (which remains to be written). Then I left.

The next day the magazine called; they wanted to publish the article. Good things were beginning to happen.

6

The Last Run

I met Roger Hartnett late one Saturday morning, and we went to the park to see how far I could "run."

I brought a fold-up cane. I was determined to go as far as I could go, any way I could go, and eventually I'd need it.

Starting off, I ran. It was hot. I kicked my legs out in front of me. Other runners went by me. I went by other runners; Roger stayed by my side. Saturday morning in Central Park, there were battalions of runners. I heard them breathing seriously, watched their shirts darkening with sweat. The runners' legs stretched and their feet beat the ground. They looked beautiful. Running, I felt beautiful, too, but I knew it wouldn't last. My ugliness was coming fast.

And it did come. The tightness in my right thigh, the toe of my left foot stubbing the ground. I stopped trying to run and began walking jerkily. Determination, Griffin. Heel down into the ground first. Foot up over the ground behind. Soon I was lurching, slowly galumphing along. Ugly. Someone to glance at as you ran past, but look away fast. You were brought up right; don't stare.

Finally Roger said something and I took the elastic off my fold-up cane and shook it straight. If anyone I knew was around, I hoped they wouldn't recognize me; I hoped they'd think I was someone else. "Someone else" careened on.

The sun was so hot. Roger talked on and on, trying to distract me, trying to keep my mind on things other than my "running," but I needed to concentrate on my complicated task.

The MS ghost hung upside down on me, its teeth sunk into my left ankle, its nails dug into my right thigh. Would it always hang like this? It was so heavy.

Roger saw a man he knew and wanted to stop and talk. The man had ropey legs and a tan. He was about twenty years older than I, sweating and puffing a bit. I balanced on my cane and stared at his sneakers. His rumpled old sneakers made me want to cry.

I could fold my shoulders together, I thought. I could become very thin, so thin nobody could see me.

Roger's friend said some polite things to me. I didn't answer him, though. I didn't intend to be rude; I just couldn't. Roger said good-bye for both of us and we went on a little farther. By this time I was crying quietly.

"Let's stop," he said suddenly. I didn't want to stop "running," though. I could go farther, I could!

"We really should stop, my building is across the street." We went to the water fountain first and I poured water all over me.

I galumphed over to Roger's building. In his apartment, I collapsed on the couch. "No, no," he said, "we're going into the kitchen." I couldn't believe I had to get up on my aching legs and galumph into the kitchen. I understood the infamous irritability of sick people then; I felt it, too. Sick people do inconvenient things and then get mad at you when you tell them not to. It's because they inconveniently hurt.

They are also inconveniently mad about all this. I

was mad at Roger, who was trying to be nice to me. He had galumphed beside me and not even broken into a sweat. How dare he. I was in extremis, or so I felt, and he wasn't even bothered. And all this pain and humiliation was his fault. He hadn't believed me when I told him how with MS, I could run fine for a little while and then would start painfully galumphing. He'd meant well; he thought he had a great new idea that I should try, that the galumphing would even off after a while and I'd be able to go on and on with just a little limp.

But the limping had gotten worse. And new things had added on to it. This is the way MS is! I told him so; why didn't he believe me? I knew it was unfair, but I hated, hated, hated him. He thought he was so smart. He thought I wasn't trying. He thought I was lazy and being easy on myself. Well, wasn't it wonderful, I'd shown him.

I couldn't stand either of us.

I tried to be pleasant as Roger's friendly wife got a six-pack of Bud out of the refrigerator. We sat around the dining-room table, talking and drinking and eating pretzels. Somebody came to join us and they were all talking and laughing, but I had a hard time joining in. I smiled at the joking while I surreptitiously made stick people with stiff legs out of my sticklike pretzels. And bit off their heads.

The isolation people who are sick talk about is partly self-imposed. Solipsism is the common denominator of all sorts of illness experiences. While other people traded jokes, I thought about myself. Just a short run—only a hop fifteen months earlier—but two and a half miles was now impossible to run. And I had become so ugly, so repellent. Hadn't regular people recoiled? Hadn't Roger's friend smiled as if I were from another world? An ugly, harmless, stupid alien, benign but gross.

What could I have done to deserve this?

I will never go "running" again, I said to myself. Never again.

Because I was with amputee Roger, I can never think that I am special. At least not because locomotion is sometimes difficult for me. It's difficult for lots of people. Being different and weird in any way—whether or not the difference is galumphing—is a painful experience. In fact, we all know something about how it feels.

I'm lucky that locomotion—walking—is not always a difficult thing for me; sometimes I forget that. I think how rotten it is that I'm so young and this has happened to me. I loved dancing and I loved sports, but this has happened to me. I exercised and took care of my health— didn't smoke, stayed thin, didn't eat lots of fats—but this has happened to me. I forget to be grateful that my MS isn't worse, that walking isn't always hard for me. At times, I forget the ways I'm lucky.

Sometimes if I'm wobbling on the street, people whisper: How much have you had to drink? Or they smile knowingly and snicker: What drugs are you on? The snickering people are cruel and wrong. I say to myself: Why should I care? I do care horribly, though.

There's a popular idea these days, that you are responsible for getting a disease. That somehow you are at fault for not being well. That positive thinking and eating right will protect you from all ills. I believe that everyone has responsibility for taking precautions—sure, we don't have to smoke or eat foods full of cholesterol. But not all illness is avoidable, and even the diseases that can be avoided are hardly their victims' fault.

In a 1978 article Ellen Goodman said it well: "As we focus on the aspects of self-health, we begin to look at all illness as self-inflicted, and even regard death as a kind of personal folly."

It's human, of course, to try to judge the victims of a disease, to make yourself somehow safe from it. "This happened to you and not to me because you are somehow different from me. You don't think right or eat right— surely you did something to bring it on yourself!"

Frankly, I don't think "eating wrong" means a disease is deserved, and I especially don't think that "thinking wrong" or experiencing negative emotions means you "brought it on yourself." Negative emotions may precipitate an attack of a disease; that's different from causing the disease, though. It's cruel folklore that so many people think these are causes.

Emotions are important, however. Positive emotions allow you to live a rich life despite having a disease and to do well even though disease darkens the horizon.

Blaming the victim has been around since way before lepers rang bells and called out, "Unclean! Unclean!" Sometimes even I want to blame this victim and claim responsibility for my MS. The positive reason behind this urge is that if I'm responsible, I might have some control of the disease.

The negative reason erupts when I accuse myself of willing this disease on myself. There are reasons why I might "choose" to have MS, especially mild MS, instead of being robustly healthy. The weakness, the being off-balance and what I consider "looking ugly" caused by MS—there are reasons why I might consider these things appropriate punishments for myself. But then I think of my cat that died of cancer, or a baby who has AIDS, and I can't believe that they are in any way responsible for their diseases. So I go back—with relief—to holding myself blameless.

I've heard that the perception of control is the most important component of a person's ability to recover, at least their psychological equilibrium, when they've had a bad time. This is certainly a sticking point for people who have things happen to them that they don't feel in control of, such as an accident that has left them disabled, or a debilitating disease.

If something bad happens that is out-of-control, there won't be much that you can do to change it. But you can always be in control, and see yourself as in control, of your thoughts, your feelings, and your behavior. In addition, any person in an out-of-control situation can look to other areas of life where he or she *is* in control for a feeling of competence and strength. Letting other things, such as your kids or your work, remind you that in some areas you do very well can help you deal better with the out-of-control part of your life. Don't let your entire life collapse because something bad happened over which you had no control.

People who use their circumstances can see themselves as doers, not as done-tos. They say, "I can't change this, but I'm going to find something good to come of it." In the final analysis, I compromise with my desire to take responsibility for having the disease and my desire to not be blamed for it. I say, "Griffin, it's not your fault that this has happened to you. But you *are* responsible for the way you live with that disease—you're responsible for learning something from it and for doing something with what you've learned."

After four years with MS, I think I have a practical and realistic attitude now, in 1988. I don't think about the disease quite so often: It's not going to overwhelm me and I'm not going to overwhelm it. Sheer willpower can't conquer it, as I once hoped. I have continued to write magazine articles and am now taking courses in biopsychology in hopes of working in the field of neuropsychology someday. I'm grateful for the physical abilities I still have, and I appreciate them in a way I never did before. When I had all my abilities intact, I was never as good as I just had to be—I was so critical of myself for not being a better climber, rider, runner, weight lifter. As if sports were so important that just enjoying them wasn't enough; I had to be good at them. Almost everything I can do now is pleasurable, just because I can do it.

Of course, exercise is important for anyone's health; it improves your looks and your mood, too. For me, it also diminishes certain changes wrought by MS—it lessens the can't-dos. Although in many ways I can't perform at a normal level, it does help maintain my current degree of physical ability. So I do run now—or, at least, race-walk for half a mile or so, on a regular basis. But now I sit down when I get tired instead of going on just to go on. I avoid becoming noticeably spastic and jerky—what's the point? I'd rather not drop from exhaustion; I have other things to do. It's pointless to spend your energy on something that isn't meaningful, so I do exercise but I also try to conserve energy and use it when it matters.

So I do exercise every day. For about nine months I didn't, and I became increasingly morose, as well as flabby. The MS started claiming more and more of my life. I feel happier and healthier now that I'm back at it. Maybe a triathlon is out of the picture for me now, but I have more interesting things to do than train for one.

I'm glad I rock-climbed and rode horses while I could. I would still like to play (and win!) at squash, but at least I used and enjoyed the abilities I had while I had them. I'll use the abilities I've got now for as long as they are here, and now really enjoy them. I plan on keeping them, too—though I know everybody's future is uncertain and, with MS, the future is even more uncertain. If my abilities go, they go, and I'll have a new kettle of fish to deal with. However, I don't expect them to. I expect to stay this way for a long time.

Nevertheless, I keep hoping that the MS will just go. *Just go!* Just disappear in the night so I can be normal and my legs can swing free again. For that not-impossible day, I have lots of plans. For that not-impossible day (in addition to reasons of vanity), I keep myself as strong as I can. I want to be ready to jump right in and enjoy it when it happens. I'll play squash and say "shot" whenever I hit the ball in a particularly devious way. Rail shots and cross-court shots and lobs. I want to *sweat* again.

Someday, in my lifetime, I believe that a restorative cure will be found and that the damage MS has done to me and to other people will be repaired. Alas, I don't think that cure will be found tomorrow. Not even next year; more likely in years.

But maybe sooner! Maybe much, much sooner!

I think of Jane Fonda. The nicest thing she ever did was to make fifty a robust and sexy time of life. Even if it does take twenty years, I can wait; it won't be too late to enjoy it. But I'll make sure I enjoy all I can right now.

Part II

LIVING A FULL LIFE

7

Doing What You Love

Adversity. Nobody likes it. But there's one thing to be said for it: It shows you what you're made of. This is how it works: Suppose you have a cat's foam-rubber ball in one hand and a kid's superball (the kind of rubber ball that bounces really high) in the other. Then you (playing the part of Adversity) toss them down. Hard.

The foam-rubber ball will have a really wimpy bounce. Very halfhearted. It will roll along the floor until it sticks somewhere—probably under the radiator or somewhere else nice and dusty. The superball, on the other hand, will bounce back high. Its energetic spring is the result of the kind of rubber it's made of.

People's resiliency differs a lot, too. You've probably noticed that some people come back stronger than ever after a crisis that's thrown them down hard. These people have learned from their trouble; it's strengthened them. Other people, however, just roll along until they find a rut that fits.

Life being what it is, we are all going to take a fall

at some point. The trick, then, is not to never fall; the trick is coming back up when you do.

———

I keep hearing that "a positive attitude" has a beneficial effect on people's health; certainly a negative attitude has a deleterious effect. But nobody can have "a good attitude" if he or she gets up in the morning and hates what has to be done that day; everybody knows if there's any excuse to go back to bed, that will make you use it. People who don't love what they do have no reason to get better or to make the most of what's been left to them. On the other hand, people who do love their work seem to thrive, even when a serious disease or condition threatens them.

My friend Berto has had juvenile diabetes since he was a kid. When he was in his twenties, the disease began to affect his vision. The disturbances were taken care of and his vision is pretty normal now, though he has difficulty seeing well at night. But although his eyes seem to be holding up pretty well, how long the good daytime vision will last is questionable.

Diabetes puts his vision at risk, and Berto is quite aware of this. Nevertheless, he has chosen to spend most of his free time taking, developing, and showing photographs. Photography is his avocation; he is passionate about it. The part of me that wants to doubt says: Is it wise to invest so much energy, attention, and emotion in something that may very well be lost to you? It's painful to lose any ability, but for an artist to lose his vision! Isn't Berto setting himself up for grief? Couldn't he have chosen something else to love doing, something not so vulnerable, something diabetes could never take from him?

Berto says, "I love photography and am fairly good at it. Suppose I had decided that pursuing it was off-limits because of the diabetes. That would have really been a loss. Life has given me enough limitations—I'm not going to give them to myself! Maybe the day will come when I won't be able to take photographs anymore, but I'll still have the satisfaction that years of taking them well will have brought me. I'll have to find something else if I can't see well enough for photography—I like jazz, so maybe something to do with that. But I'll worry about that when it happens."

It's self-punishing to look for activities that are particularly vulnerable if a disease progresses (though probably we all do it to some extent—nothing is so important as something you might lose). However, it's also very self-limiting to avoid those activities, especially if they mean a lot to you. I hope that Berto's vision will never be seriously impaired. I suspect that its loss, and with it the loss of photography, would be more painful to him than he cares to think about right now.

Berto does what he loves doing. That makes living and staying well very valuable to him. Everyone should do what he or she loves, since we've all got a limited life-span and as far as I know, no one gets another. Yet it may be even more important for people with diseases or conditions that limit them to do what they love, either in their jobs or as a hobby in their free time.

People do seem to gravitate toward using abilities that are "at risk." Sometimes this is wise; sometimes not. I think of it as the get-it-while-you-can attitude. I have some doubts about the wisdom of Berto's choice, but I admire his refusal to anticipate a disability that might never happen, or might not happen for many years, and limit himself accordingly. That's the bravest way to live.

Toni Phelan is pretty brave, too. She gave up an impressive income to do what she loves. Instead of analyzing communication systems, she jumps out of airplanes. For fun.

Toni insists it isn't courage, it isn't discipline: It's love that makes her skydive. In 1974, just before her first parachute jump, she went blind in one eye. The diagnosis was optic neuritis, and in a year she went blind in the other eye. Fortunately, the vision in the second eye returned after Toni was hospitalized and received a dose of steroids. But she's remained blind on one side.

Toni says, "When I was diagnosed with optic neuritis [sometimes, but not always, a precursor of MS], I decided that here was a risk I could not control. But skydiving was a risk I *could* control. If anything could have made me want to skydive more than I already did, losing vision in one eye was it. I felt that since I could still skydive now, I'd better do it. When the first eye went blind, I didn't tell my skydiving instructor for fear that I wouldn't be allowed to jump. Having only one sighted eye does disturb my depth perception—which matters in skydiving only when you're hurtling down toward people and you need to judge how far away they are and how long it will take you to get there! So I am perhaps slightly more cautious about when I choose to jump than someone who has no physical problems; I don't want to take a chance with my life or anyone else's. But there are no big changes in my jumping that I've made because of the deficit."

Toni teaches jumping now. She left her tedious but high-paying job to teach skydiving because, she says, "Jumping is such a rush! Sure, I worry about the money and medical benefits I might need someday, but I don't think about it too much. What I do now is so exciting, it's addictive. I love it."

Though Toni is slow to credit the love of her new occupation with the stability in her health (she hasn't had another attack), she says that doing what she loves makes her life meaningful and fun. She doesn't brood about the optic neuritis, but she hopes it never takes away the sport she's come to love so much.

Lillian was diagnosed with the serious autoimmune disease systemic lupus erythematosus ten years ago, when she was in her early thirties—though she thinks her first attack was almost fifteen years earlier.

SLE, or lupus, is a chronic, inflammatory, occasionally fatal disease in which the body makes antibodies that attack its own tissues. Just about any organ can be the site of a lupus attack, and the symptoms are often vague and shifting, making diagnosis a tricky undertaking. Lillian, for example, had low-grade fevers, chronic and exasperating fatigue, and odd aches and pains.

Like other autoimmune diseases, lupus seems to have a prediliction for females. Sore joints are one of its more frequent manifestations, and lupus that concentrates in the joints is often confused with rheumatoid arthritis—in fact, that's the diagnosis given to the severe chest pains emanating from her rib cage that caused Lillian to be hospitalized during her adolescence. Now, however, she suspects that they were an early symptom of lupus.

And because the sun often brings on attacks, people with lupus frequently coat themselves with sunscreens and wear voluminous clothing all summer long. This used to be a real hassle, Lillian says, but now no one gets a dark tan because the sun is known to be bad for everyone, so pale skin in the summer doesn't brand her as "different." The most characteristic symptom of the disease, however, is a "butterfly rash" that spreads over the bridge of the nose and up and down the cheeks. Even this symptom occurs in only 40 percent of patients. Lillian had the rash on only one side of her face.

When Lillian was diagnosed, she was involved in a business with a friend. They sold maternity sport clothes, and the business had really taken off. Lillian had a little girl by then and she was busy, successful, but bored.

After working to get the business off the ground, Lillian was no longer really interested. She started getting sick a lot—the low-grade fevers, mysterious aches and pains, and unremitting fatigue that, after several doctors, finally led to her being diagnosed with a frightening-sounding, sometimes fatal, and incurable disease: lupus, the rapacious wolf. After a period of flailing about and grieving, Lillian did some serious soul-searching and decided that if her life wasn't going to be as long as she'd expected (we now know lupus doesn't always shorten the life-span), then she wouldn't waste any of it doing things that "didn't matter." She came up with three articles of faith:

1. In order to be happy and make your life seem worthwhile, you need to love what you do.

2. This may involve stress, and stress has been shown to be bad for you. But there are two kinds of stress—good stress (which makes you productive) and bad stress (which drains your energy).

3. The mind has some control over anything that happens in the body. It's important to access that control in order to fight a disease.

Lillian didn't love what she was doing. So why do it? she said. She sold her part of the business and began to hunt about for some way to use her entrepreneurial skills. Starting a business (she already had two) was lots of fun, she thought. While she was casting about, she saw an ad in a little local newspaper for horseback riding lessons. She thought she'd have fun trying that. Being outside in the sunlight and pushing on her tender knee joints was probably no good for her, but she wanted to try it anyhow. So she did. She just made sure she didn't tell her doctor.

Wow! She loved horseback riding. Before you know it, she was quite a rider. She describes herself as "a natural." "Something happened when I rode—the physical connection with the animal made me happy and the happiness lessened my lupus symptoms or made them seem to go away." Soon Lillian owned two horses. Then her daughter started riding. She needed a smaller horse. Lillian was accumulating horses and expenses, and decided that this was what she loved to do. Stabling horses and starting a riding school would be her next business.

"I decided that the riding and starting the school fell under the heading of good stress," she says. "It's a difficult and anxiety-provoking business, but working with the animals is soothing and pleasurable. The hours fly by when I'm working at the stable. It's hard work but it's good stress because it's all worth it.

"Learning about horses was easy because it was fascinating. Taking care of the animals and seeing that they had good surroundings was actually a pleasure—well, it's not a pleasure to get up at night for a sick animal, but the work always seems purposeful.

"I thought my doctor would disapprove of my riding but all he said was: Whatever you're doing, keep doing it, it's working." The lupus, which still gives her achey joints and keeps her wearing sunblock, seemed to go into remission and bothered her far less.

Having a business that revolved around horses was doing what she loved. And though she can't explain how, Lillian's sure that it helped her with her disease. The lupus has never since been as virulent as it was before the new business. So two of her articles of faith—doing what she loved and having only good stress—were fulfilled by the career change to horses. The third one—using the mind to influence the body—was something else Lillian was working on.

Lillian looks great and feels great now, even though lupus had once made her very sick. If doing what you love can be this powerful an Rx, we'd all better find it.

Lillian's hard work made a difference, but not everybody's does. Some people work very hard for a very long time—with excellent results. But other people who work hard and seem just as driven and ambitious do not have their efforts rewarded. If one does not improve, however, it should not be because of not trying. It should be only because there are physical limitations on the improvement possible.

It's not a failure not to improve. Failure is not the inability to "conquer" the disease or debilitating condition; failure is not to try. When you don't try and you allow your life to dwindle because of a disease or a condition, you've resigned yourself to letting it "win."

Granted, it's often hard to tell the difference between

the stubborn refusal to quit and futilely banging your head against the wall. Only long-term results really tell you which you're doing. In the meantime, however, some guidelines can help you distinguish between determination (good) and not letting go (bad), and between acceptance (good) and resignation (bad).

Determination is doing those boring exercises day after day if you have a disease where they might make a difference, or watching your diet and insulin intake—doing whatever is required to take care of yourself. Determination means you take care of yourself and insist that your life counts. To whom? Why, to you, of course.

Not letting go, on the other hand, means you live in the past, not the present. Life in your present condition does not seem worth it to you anymore. Unless some magic makes you the same as you were, or the elusive cure turns up, you are going back to bed. Everybody probably feels that way some of the time. The trick is to not feel that way most of the time.

When you've accepted the disease, you don't try to do things that are out of reach for you now—but you love yourself and value the things you can do. With some people this means depreciating the activities that have had to go, at least for a while—go ahead, if it makes you feel better. This seems like a case of sour grapes, but if it works for you, so what?

For example, I've had to give up the idea of doing a triathlon. This ambition did not go easily, but eventually I did let go of it and now it looks almost funny—me, with my nose in a book all day, do a triathlon? Muscle-heads do triathlons. (This isn't always true, of course—I knew a man in medical school who did a triathlon.) Not only could I not finish one, but the training seems like an awful waste of time. I have better things to do now. I've changed my values and accepted the fact that an amateur athlete, I'm not.

Resignation, on the other hand, can be the same as giving up. It's not making the most of the abilities you do have. Not only do you want it all back (which is reasonable), but you refuse to live with what you've got. You just wait for the cure, which has proven to be damned elusive.

Most people are defeated not by a problem but by a lack of imagination. The ability to shift focus and use an alternate route is a hallmark of people who come back strong. They have often found a different way to reach their goal that incorporates the new set of circumstances. By using their imaginations, they see more than a problem; they also see a possibility. People who think "there's only one way to do it" balk at an unexpected obstacle and can't go on.

People who don't get stuck in stressful situations but go on to other things are comfortable taking tributaries and changing horses in the middle of a stream. The goal, after all, is getting to the other side, not getting there in any particular way.

Dealing with smaller troubles is "practice" for dealing with major catastrophes. People who've had lucky and well-protected lives are likely to feel overwhelmed by a crisis. People who've had "practice" are more likely to look at trouble as a normal, if unpleasant, part of life. They deal with it (which includes feeling bad about it) and get on with living—instead of rehashing it over and over and wondering why it happened to them.

When people cope with adversity, they strengthen their coping abilities for the future, psychologists say. Because they've dealt with adversity before, they know that they're able to survive it, that they aren't going to fall apart. Resiliency is something that you learn.

Everyone has despairing moments. It's impossible to always have a positive outlook when your body is threatened; however, having a positive outlook most of the time *is* possible, and is what you can shoot for.

8

Family and Friends

I have an imposter complex. I go around appearing normal a lot of the time, but we know the truth. Sometimes I feel the real me is simply incognito when I appear all right. The real me has a laborious, unsexy, old person's walk. She doesn't always show, but I'd have to live a very constricted life for the real me to never show: no long walks in the park because then she might come out; no aerobic anything where people might see me. The real me is the awkward, clumsy, hard-for-me-to-love me. I take cabs sometimes to keep her from coming out: The walk to and from a subway stop might be too far to do "normally." The real me might show.

Often, though, I let her show. It's sad to limp and be uncoordinated, to have to hang on to someone for balance, but it's sadder to be alone.

More often than before, I am alone. Sometimes it's my choice. Sometimes I just can't do what other people are doing; sometimes I can, at least in a way, but I would feel so awkward. I try to make sure that I'm by myself when I'm most disabled. I think it's like wearing your oldest bathrobe only when you're alone. It's easy and relaxed, but you'd rather other people didn't see you in it.

I take exercise or dance classes when I have the time. Even though they always make me look weird, they are just too good for me to forgo. I explain that I have MS to the teachers; otherwise they get scared when the symptoms start to show. They think: This must be an emergency! Something is happening to her! What am I supposed to do?

I stand in the back row. (I always think of that board game I played as a kid when I take my position in the back row. It was called Go to the Head of the Class. But just when you were about to be the first one finished and win the game, you'd land on a square that said Go to the Bottom of the Class and you'd have to start all over. That's how I feel when I take a position in the back row.)

All those years when I would "demonstrate" an exercise or a dance move, trying not to look like I was loving it, trying not to look like I was showing off a bit. Who me, show off? Never! My ego wasn't massaged by "demonstrating." Not at all! Now I go to the back row, so as not to alarm other students, so as not to be stared at by them.

There must be an easier way to learn that a talent is good luck and hard work, not some kind of superiority and hard work. Did I really deserve to be good then? Do I really deserve to be bad now? Oh, well. Just do it if you can do it, Griffin.

Because I swing through such a wide range—sometimes I seem normal (I'm actually off-balance or ataxic all the time; if you're looking for it, you can see it) and sometimes clearly disabled—it's hard for anybody, including myself, to have a clear idea of "the real me." Though sometimes I think of the real me as being crippled (at least, when I'm in a bad mood), most of the time I think of the real me as being able to jump tall buildings in a single bound. The onset of the slowness, the jerkiness and incoordination (that is, the galumphing) is not quite as surprising as it used to be, but when it descends, I still feel that I've become a stranger, someone else.

There are positive aspects to being apparently disabled only part of the time. One is obvious: I don't always go through the pain of disability; sometimes I can almost forget it. The second good thing is that I have a special window on how healthy people treat the ill. People treat me one way when they think that I'm okay; they treat me differently when they see that I'm not "normal."

When I'm disabled, people's faces turn to masks. Their voices become syrupy. They try to hide their pity and fear but the masks say as much as the naked feelings would. And maybe naked feelings would convey more respect; the masks say, I know you can't take this, the fact of what you are. You unfortunate thing. I'm glad that I'm not you.

I remind them of something they'd rather forget— the mortality and human vulnerability we have in common. They look worried. Suppose I fall and hurt myself; what will they do? I make them uneasy.

They make *me* uneasy. On their faces I read what I don't want to be true: I do look strange, I am vulnerable, my mortality is showing, I might fall and hurt myself.

I know most people are really sympathetic, but they're also scared and don't know how to react. I don't always know how I want people to react, either. I want to be treated normally—even though I'm not normal. I want my problems to be acknowledged—even though I want them to be ignored. You'd have to be a genius to figure out what I really want.

I guess I'm still uncomfortable with the fact of the MS, and I don't know what I want because my needs change all the time. Anyway, the discomfort is my problem. People who are normal shouldn't worry about it.

Not everyone puts on a mask. And since I'm still frequently defensive about the MS, I misunderstand genuine kindness at times. For example, last week a bus driver said, "You've had a hard time. The ride's on me," and gave me back my fare. I don't think he was being patronizing; he was just being nice. Once I would have felt belittled. (Okay. He was being nice, but I also liked getting my money back.)

With some outstanding exceptions, it's less painful for me to be with new friends now who don't realize how much I've changed. And it's less painful to new friends to be with me. They aren't shocked at the new me; they don't —ugh—feel sorry for me. Some friends (maybe I mean acquaintances, not friends) look appalled when my limitations become apparent to them; they hug me good-bye with so much fervor I'm embarrassed, then don't return my calls. When I went to a party at Martin's (an old rock-climbing friend), I had to ask him to help me step up and climb out a window onto his back porch. (Yes, he's a New Yorker. Even though the porch is hard to get to, his place is considered really great.) This is something any normal person could do without help; a rock climber should navigate this route with ease. But I couldn't; I needed help.

Martin did help, but he looked at me so strangely first. Then at the end of the party, he hugged me good-bye so strongly, so oddly, I wondered why. Yeah, he's one who stopped returning my calls; other people told me why. ("He said he just can't stand it.") Well, he's not the only one. Maybe MS did kill the old Moira; then may she rest in peace. A new Moira has taken over, and, believe me, she has no time for someone as fragile as rock-climber Martin.

I think I understand why some people act like he did, but in no way do I excuse them. I can't be included in the things they like to do anymore. And I stir up fear in them; after all, what's happened to me could happen to them. So they just can't stand it.

But some old friends hang in there. They make you feel so loved just by including you, considering you. They value something about you that hasn't changed. Even if you can't do the same old things, they help you find something else you can enjoy together. Even if it's just going to the movies.

Old friends like that aren't floored by misfortune. They don't like what's happened, but they really think about you and what you can do now. For example, just when I was about to let a big part of me die—in this case, the me that liked adventurous sports so much—just when I was about to throw in the towel and say there's *nothing! nothing!* that I can do like that anymore, an old friend called me with a perfect solution.

I was in the slough of despond thinking of all the things I loved that I'd probably never do again, when Jeannie (another rock climber) called one night. "Moira! I thought of something that's just right for you. Scuba!" Since I no longer think of myself as a very physical person, I sighed, thinking how Jeannie would not let the old me go. But a few weeks later, I thought, Scuba! What a great idea! Swimming is something I'm good at. Cold water makes this even more appealing, and you can't fall down in the water. I called Jeannie back and thanked her.

I haven't tried scuba yet, but I'm going to. It's expensive, but I'll figure out some way to afford it.

And now that I'm back at school, I have something else to share with friends who have similar, though not exactly the same, interests. Neuropsychology, what I'm interested in, is related to cognitive psychology, and since I have a couple of friends who are involved in that, our friendships have shifted and now we share that interest instead of athletics.

And people who've known me since I was a kid love me for a reason that has nothing to do with any of the physical things I counted on for so long. Those things really don't seem like such important qualities any more. What do these people love me for? Well, that ineffable thing, me-ness, I suppose.

Anyone making a similar, unwanted transition in his or her life will find the same things hold true: Some people who are only associated with a certain lost activity may indeed no longer be friends. Other friendships will shift their focus. But the oldest and dearest friends will stick with you come hell or high water. They love you for a reason beyond shared activities, beyond shared interests.

Your best and oldest friends are probably your family. This isn't true for everybody, but for many people it is. They understand your anger. They probably are angry, too, that life has done this to you.

It's a relief to be able to let the angry feelings out—they are normal to anyone who's taken a blow from life—and not feel disliked for them. Most other people don't want to share the burden of intense and angry feelings; it's too much for them. They aren't close enough to you to want to be bothered. It is a bother, and they've got their own problems. But most members of a family will understand your feelings, feel them with you, validate them, even feel you're entitled to them. You deserve to be angry; they're angry, too.

A loving family won't want you to get stuck there. Besides being angry, there are other things for you to do. They will remember this, even if you're temporarily swamped by the notion of loss. Whatever you've lost, you are still *you*. Since your family continues loving you no matter what, you're reminded that your most lovable, most essential qualities have little to do with what you've lost. This won't make you happy about your situation, but it can help cut the panic a bit.

The most difficult—and probably the most common—situation involves the overprotective family or parent. It's always hard to resist letting people do things for you and it's especially hard when the person is your parent. But that situation is in nobody's best interest.

When a parent is overprotective, it probably feels and is overcontrolling. Most likely, they are trying to assuage irrational guilt: somehow they should have protected you from this! So they'll do their protecting now. But MS rarely means that a person is no longer able to care for her- or himself. Parents and family are helpful when emotional support is needed; but they should know when to let go, too.

Often they don't. And it's often hard for the MS person to tell when interest in his or her life becomes interference in his or her life.

Self-esteem is often based upon taking care of oneself, however. Of course, a person with any chronic disease should take care of his- or herself as much as possible. Talking openly with parents and other family members is probably the only way to prevent or stop overprotectiveness.

Not every family is a haven. Even if they don't mean to, your spouse or siblings and parents might inadvertently make a bad situation worse. Because family members are involved in the outcome of any problem that affects you, they may not be as helpful as someone who is more objective and uninvolved.

It is very human to let the "bearer of bad tidings" suffer the brunt of the anger his tidings have caused. (In ancient Greece, didn't they slaughter the bearer of bad tidings? So direct with their feelings, those Greeks.) In many situations, you will be the bearer. So, not only will your family be angry for you, they will also be a little angry at you. For example, I have received a lot of support and consolation from my family. But since MS occurs with slightly higher frequency in families, my three sisters have a higher than average risk of also getting the disease. (The risk is still very small, however. Most likely they will be fine.) The higher chance of it affecting them, though, is made clear by me—though I didn't make their risk higher, I'm proof that it is. In a way, I'm the bearer of bad tidings for them. It's reasonable to assume there's a little resentment on their part.

This is only one example of the fact that anything that affects you affects the people closest to you. They can't help but have expectations for you and of you. A family member's feelings of resentment and anger at a person who has become dependent, and his or her guilt because something that happened to another member "should have happened to him or her," are irrational, but human. Still, they can make matters worse. And the hurt person secretly, or not so secretly, wishing it had happened to anybody else is normal and human; not so nice, but ordinary.

Nobody's feelings are pure. If yours are, I guess you're not human. What this means, though, is sometimes your feelings are more easily vented outside the family.

If that's the case, create a "family" that will fulfill your needs. Many people use support groups for this purpose. Even if your own family is supportive, it can help to have other people who really understand what you're going through because they've been there themselves, and who won't have anything invested in dealing with the crisis in a certain way.

Two people I respect a lot—my friends Jane and Lillian—recommend support groups very highly. Jane's second daughter, Rachel, was born blind, and she also has seizures and is mentally retarded. Jane, of course, is brokenhearted. The mother of a child born with any handicap undergoes many complicated and painful feelings—irrational guilt, as well as anger and sorrow, feelings that are difficult to understand for anyone who hasn't had a similar experience. But in the support group she joined, specifically for mothers of handicapped children, she could let her feelings out and feel understood.

Only the mothers in Jane's support group seemed to understand what the long months of waiting to be sure that the child wasn't intellectually normal meant to Jane, and how wildly she wanted Rachel to be one of the handful of lucky ones. And her new grief when it slowly became apparent that she wasn't.

Jane's family had different ways of dealing with

Rachel's problem. They wanted to find another doctor, as if another doctor could change the facts. Their denial was an added frustration for Jane. In the support group, she felt understood.

My friend Lillian—the woman who has lupus but runs a horseback riding business—never joined a group specifically for people with a chronic disease, but has been involved in group therapy for many years. She feels that by confronting and accepting your feelings, you keep them from manifesting themselves in your body. Feelings are wily, Lillian says, and if you refuse to recognize and express them, they'll come out in some way—in her case, unexpressed feelings might aggravate inflamed joints or organs. She credits the therapy group with her education in recognizing suppressed emotion, and she credits this ability of hers in part with her long remission.

I've always felt a little apprehensive about joining a group for people with MS—I thought it would make me identify with the disease too much. I want MS to be as small a part of my life as it can be. But I have participated in groups in which people have various disabilities, and this has been very good for me. For one thing, it reminded me that having physical problems and disabilities was not so unique. And that, compared to many others, my situation was not so bad. It helped me take my mind off myself and become more compassionate. Also, because I met people I liked in these groups and people I was sure were in no way accountable for their handicaps, it made me realize in a deep way what was apparent from the start—I wasn't responsible for getting a disease, and I didn't get it because I deserved it.

It's a very human characteristic, I think, to try to explain things, and it's so convenient to explain diseases and disabilities by thinking that in some way their victims are at fault; they deserved what they got. Since there's no clear biological explanation yet for MS, or for many other diseases, such as cancer, it's even easier to think of some metaphysical reason for it. If society were only a little more primitive, we'd have no problem saying that spirits did it. MS is such a weird disease, you can almost believe that. But don't. It does you no good to feel in any way culpable for a disease or condition. But I do believe that you are responsible for living the best life with it that you can.

9

Sex and Disability

Sexuality doesn't stop when a person becomes disabled, but it changes for most people. Especially for most single people. It certainly changed for me, and it is still hard to talk about.

The change in my sexuality isn't "physical." Like most young people with multiple sclerosis, my sexual function is unchanged. According to the *Multiple Sclerosis Fact Book* by Richard Lechtenberg, M.D., young people especially should check for other possible causes of sexual dysfunction: that is, pain during intercourse, lack of vaginal lubrication, impotence, or sexual disinterest. There are other possible physical reasons for sexual problems. One should eliminate them before assuming that the problems are caused by MS.

However, while MS might not always affect sexual function, at times it does. According to Lechtenberg, as many as half the women and about 25 to 40 percent of the men with MS between eighteen and fifty report a change in their sexual response. This is usually due to lack of vaginal lubrication in females, or lack of erection and ejaculation in males. But sometimes spasticity causes the disruption by making common positions difficult, or by constricting the vaginal opening, making penetration painful for either party. Sometimes there is a lack of orgasm in either partner, or even a lack of desire.

Some of these problems can be solved. For example, if the problem is lack of vaginal lubrication, lubricants are available for purchase. If the problem relates to spasticity in the limbs, different positions, or an antispasticity drug, can be tried. If the problem is lack of desire on the affected person's part, however, it will be more complicated to deal with. A therapist familiar with the problems associated with MS can be helpful in treating this.

For most young people, however, I don't know that those disabilities are the crux of the problem. They are sad and do limit the ways some people can have sex, but there are unorthodox ways to have sex or be "physical" with someone, ways that range from hugging to using a penile prosthesis or an unusual position in bed—whatever works for you and your partner. I don't mean to belittle those problems or to pretend that any of the solutions offered are ideal, but I firmly believe that if you really want to please someone sexually, you can.

Therefore, there is no real reason to think that a disability prevents you from being a good sexual partner. But I think a fear that you're undesirable is crippling sexually. It's certainly a feeling that can still grip me.

It's a lack of self-esteem that makes me feel I'm undesirable. (That, and an uncool former male friend.) I remind myself that I can still wrap my legs around a special person and be very happy. I remind myself that certain people do find me desirable and let me know. So why do I persist in feeling this way?

Common sense says that feeling undesirable, especially when presented with evidence to the contrary, probably predates the multiple sclerosis. But I think that even if that worry has always been there, MS exacerbated it. MS also made the feeling of being undesirable seem more believable by limiting the activities I could engage in where I might meet someone to become intimate with. And if someone did seem to desire me, I could rather easily dismiss it, figuring that "well, he just doesn't know." If he got close to me, he would have to know. And I thought then I'd be "dumped." Because, after all, even with a small disability, I couldn't be desirable. How could I convince myself that I was wrong?

I asked able-bodied and disabled people (including myself): Can a disabled person be sexually attractive to you? Some of the feedback I got was heartening; some was dismaying. The most "honest" answers were inadvertent—and they were, predictably, mixed. I will never forget them, though. Even when MS becomes a thing of the past—as someday it will, as someday it must—I'll remember those answers.

One of the hardest things about having any disability is feeling unattractive. And MS often hits in the early adult years when feeling attractive seems so important. And it's the unsurprising truth that a disabled person is not attractive to some people simply because of the fact of the disability. Those people aren't everybody; nevertheless, I've talked to a lot of people, and I have concluded that although disability doesn't make one unlovable, it does make it harder to find a lover. And the difficulty increases with the degree of disability. (But it's always hard to find a lover who matters, my sensible self reminds me.)

Nevertheless, it's a tough row to hoe. You can't change yourself if you want to be more attractive when the unattractive thing is disability. You can plan on losing weight when the unattractive thing is too much weight, or on quitting smoking if you think that will do it. Those are changes that you can make, even if they are often difficult; you are in control. Knowing that you can't make the change, knowing that you're not in control, is damned hard.

For a while, then, it's all right to just be sad about it. Desirability is another loss, and it deserves to be mourned. Being sad is appropriate; being out-of-control is hard to bear, even hard to acknowledge. While I was in this period I thought a lot about how I used to rely on looks, and might have thought they were more important than they were. Well, in some ways they are important. They do attract positive attention. People seem to think that beautiful equals good and healthy. Neither is always true, but because of this equation, I never think it's silly that some people spend so much time trying to improve their looks. Appearance can have a real effect on people's attitude toward you. Having good looks doesn't mean you'll be spared anything, though. I'm still me, whether I look good or absolutely awful.

Despite knowing this, I worry about my looks a lot. Every little line on my face is a cause for panic. I see gray hair on my head and think nobody will love me. And then when the MS acts up, I still think "Oh, give up."

I saw a book of poetry with a wonderful title: *The End of Beauty*. I think the poet was referring to a change that occurs in some artists' work as they and their work mature: The work loses its beauty. Beautiful images, sounds, even thoughts are deleted in favor of stuff that is real and truthful—material that is powerful but not beautiful.

In my life, beauty tends to refer to the usual sort of thing considered female beauty for American women— big eyes, slim hips, all that. I've been pretty, but once I liked to think maybe I could be beautiful. Since I also was athletic (and intolerably proud of it) I thought that I had a version of male beauty, too—physical prowess.

I think that's why most of us want to be good-looking. We think we could attract the opposite sex more easily if only we were beautiful. Maybe women even felt, deep down, that they'd be safer, be taken care of. Men seem to jump through flaming hoops for beautiful women, I thought; doors open automatically.

But beauty is a pretty flimsy thing to base your hopes on. I know feminists have been saying this for years; I have said it all my life. But did I really believe it? I certainly didn't make any provisions for life without good looks.

One day when I was walking home after seeing my analyst, I gradually changed from normal to spastic. I passed an old guy sitting on an orange crate in a store front. He had made vulgar remarks to me once before when I'd walked past looking normal. This time, as I limped past, he said gently, "Angel, how ya doin?"

I suppose I should have felt "See, he's not so bad." But instead I had to hold back the tears—he pitied me! A line from a poem I wrote in college went round and round in my head: sexless as an angel. Sexless as an angel.

I spent a lot of time trying to be sexy and attractive because I thought I wasn't anymore.

So what! I'm not sexy or attractive when I'm spastic and uncoordinated. I'm still the same, and yet I'm so changed.

When I'm "normal," I feel normal—maybe happy, maybe sad, but not connected to MS—but when I'm galumphing I feel angry, sorry for myself, and scared. If I galumphed all the time I'd probably learn to feel normal-for-me when I was that way, but because it's occasional (though not infrequent), I still feel intensely bad. I always wonder if it means I'm getting worse, and I still feel scared and furious. (I'd nevertheless take occasional rather than constant galumphing, any time.) At times I still think everything that goes wrong in my life is because of MS. There are far worse things, I know, and I also know that most people have *something* wrong with them—either physical or psychological. I'm still *Moira*, no matter what!

I decided to talk to Jill, a woman who is not beautiful in the conventional sense, but who is beautiful in other ways, ways I'd like to emulate. She's a disabled person whose life is full, romantically and otherwise, and who is extremely successful professionally. Jill had polio myelitis as a child and gets around in a motorized wheelchair. She has a good job and is dedicated to helping other disabled people. When I went to see her, I danced around the question I really wanted to ask. I was afraid it was rude for someone so much less disabled to ask: What about disability and feeling unattractive?

I watched her at her office dialing the phone with a mouthstick. Her hands were puffy with edema—she couldn't use them—but she had long, painted nails. Who painted her nails—her kids? And how long did her manicures last if she never used her hands?

Jill was married and had two children she had borne herself. They were fine. Her husband stayed home and took care of the children—Jill had an advanced degree and could earn more working than he could. The two little kids probably needed his physical abilities, too.

How did she meet her husband? I asked. Through a job she'd had, she answered. (How normal! I thought.) It was at a community place, years ago. Kids came there after school to play pool or shoot baskets, and she checked out the balls for them. Her husband did something like that there, too. It wasn't an immediate attraction (she smiled at me) but it grew into a compelling one.

Sometimes her kids fed her now, she said. (What unusual and interesting people they were going to grow up to be, I thought.) In general, her husband did all of the child-care chores. Clearly, you aren't guaranteed to meet someone like him; but it's guaranteed that you won't if you always stay home.

I also wondered about the "unattractiveness" of the anger that festered in me—and in other disabled people. She has to be angry, I thought. People only a few years older than I had not had the polio vaccine, including Jill. Polio was epidemic when I was a child, and many, alas, had polio myelitis when they were just kids. Polio is a virus that attacks the motor nerves of the spinal cord, and the resulting disability range is wide.

"Aren't you angry that so little effort was made to help the people who had had polio after the vaccine stopped its spread?" I asked Jill. She didn't say anything, so I added, "I worry that a vaccine to prevent MS will be discovered and nobody will care about the disease getting worse in the people who already have it: So what, they're only 250,000 Americans." (Generally, I consider this an irrational worry, for all sorts of reasons.) Postpolio syndrome, a progressive weakening of the still-innervated muscles, had recently been identified in polio survivors who had become adults. After years, their little bit of muscle innervation started wearing out.

"Aren't you angry?" I asked her again.

"Yes," she answered curtly.

So she is angry, but the rest of her life seems to go on beautifully. Anger isn't as much of a problem to me as it used to be. Once you understand it, identify with it, and also realize it's not directed at you, it seems far more benign. I can't quite understand why anger used to seem so frightening. Now I just wish there was less reason for it.

After talking to Jill, I thought, I certainly complain a lot, having so much less than she to complain about. Jill is an inspiring person; she does so much with so little that she proves you've got no excuse. And with a demanding job, a husband, and two terrific kids, her life certainly is not "on hold."

Sexuality certainly doesn't have to be given up, but newly restricted abilities may mean a change in how you meet people. Many singles' activities are athletic, and many put emphasis on attracting someone through the way you look. For obvious reasons, these activities probably will not help someone with anything more serious than a very mild disability. However, "normal" people as well as disabled people tend to build friendships with members of the opposite sex before becoming involved in deep romantic relationships. For people interested in developing a relationship, meeting people at work and participating in activities such as continuing education, volunteer work, or community action are ways to meet others with the same interests. For the mildly impaired, of course, nonaerobic sports, dancing, and so on are still viable ways to meet people.

Don't care about just anybody's opinion—that's practically a prescription for getting hurt. Choose carefully whose opinion counts. You probably heard something like that from your mother when you were about ten. Well, she was right. Value yourself in lots of ways, and value yourself as a sexual partner even though some people might not be able to think of you that way.

It's terribly important to learn whose opinion is worth taking to heart. A lot of people have foolish or cruel opinions and values, but not everybody. Nevertheless, sometimes it doesn't seem easy to find someone to appreciate you, and it seems awfully hard to ignore the ones who don't.

I wasn't going out with anybody in the spring of 1988, and I wondered if it was because of the MS. I thought my "best" friend, Phillip, who had known me for years, would happily reassure me. I needed him to.

Phillip had seen me at my worst. He had seen how MS could disable me, he had even seen me fall down. And he had seen me looking normal. I was counting on him to say that the MS didn't matter; that I was still attractive, that what was inside was what counted. Of course, some man would desire and love me. I should have given him the script. But I thought he wouldn't need prompting; I thought he could say all this sincerely.

We were friends. We talked on the phone a lot, shared books and spaghetti suppers, listened to 1970s rock and roll. We'd been friends for nine years and had even taken a trip around Vermont on our bicycles together. Which is just to explain why I thought Phillip would consider any man lucky to call himself mine. I figured he appreciated my "deeper self"; I thought I appreciated his.

I called him. I asked him if he thought I was still desirable. His answer was basically "no."

He told me to look for a lover who was disabled. It was all over for me with normal people. "Phillip! Sometimes I find a disabled person attractive—you know about

George—but are you telling me to confine myself to them? That nobody 'normal' would have me now? That damaged goods are worthy only of damaged goods?'' I said after a moment. "Phillip! Is that what you're saying?''

"I don't want to protect you," he said.

Temporarily, I believed him. I cried. I swore vengeance. Someday, somehow, I'd make Phillip desire me, then turn him down.

Wallowing in misery, I wondered if I should quit now. Self-slaughter. It would be a way of maintaining dignity and some control; putting the period at the end of a life sentence. If there was only humiliation, suffering, and incapacity to come, if I was going to become asexual and a burden to those who once loved me, maybe I should quit now.

My roommate had a little safe in her closet that she never locked and in which she kept her prescription drugs. I took a bottle or two of Dalmane from there. Dalmane is a kind of sleeping pill that comes in red-and-yellow capsules. I lined the capsules up in a row and looked at them. I stared at them. Did I want to die?

Now it seems a ridiculous question to ask myself, because the answer was obvious—I wanted to live. So what if Phillip said that I was not desirable? Desirability is hardly the only reason to live. Then, however, being undesirable seemed unbearable.

Besides, I don't really believe I'm undesirable. Maybe to some people I am. But I can deal with that, can't I?

Maybe in some cockeyed way, I was thinking about getting back at Phillip. Having my death on his conscience ought to make him feel bad! But it would make me feel even worse. I started to get mad.

Suicide: capital punishment of the self. If someone had disabled me, capital punishment might be just right for them. (At least so I irrationally think.) But who had done this to me? I certainly hadn't. Why was I angry at myself? Why was I thinking of punishing myself? I wanted to get well, not die.

I didn't know that I'd get worse. I might not. I should

stick around and find out. Suppose I killed myself and
the cure was found next year. The way I was was not
unbearable. Getting worse would not be unbearable. And
there were still a lot of things I wanted to do.

The first thing I wanted to do was quickly dis-
patched. I wrote Phillip a letter (while humming the Bea-
tles tune about being crippled inside). I said I didn't think
we should be friends anymore.

It was late; I went to bed. The next morning I swept
the pills back into the bottle and pressed down the cap.
How sophomoric. The self-pity was gross, maudlin. It
belittled the reasons that people really wanted to die. Was
the sleeping-pill drama some morbid entertainment for
me? I don't know, but I hadn't even taken one.

Telling Phillip that I didn't want to be his friend anymore
was painful after nine years. I still miss him, but I think
it was an important and positive move on my part. Don't
keep people around who are negative and who hurt you;
protect yourself from them. You deserve friends who will
do you good—you can do them good. "Friends" like
Phillip will probably say they are just being honest; what
a way to hide that they are just being cruel!

Despite thinking that letting go of Phillip was a good
move, I knew that during our little interchange I had lost
a lot: a person I thought was my friend, as well as the
notion of myself as attractive and sexy. It was something
I'd always counted on; too much, no doubt, but still. I
knew being attractive wasn't a reason for anyone to love
you, but I thought it might be a reason why someone
might want to get to know you. This was right around
the time when *Newsweek* and other publications were de-
livering the doleful news of the infamous Harvard study:
Very few women in their thirties could expect to marry.
I was thirty-three, and I wanted to be married. If I accepted Phillip's opinion, I may as well forget it.

Maybe Phillip's bad news referred only to himself.
So what if he wasn't attracted to me? I wasn't attracted
to him. I knew some disabled people who didn't seem

to be doing too badly with the opposite sex. Jill, for example, and how about single Beth? Maybe I should talk to her. I called Beth.

Beth is a pretty and intelligent woman in her late twenties who is in a wheelchair. She's popular and outgoing, cheerful and funny. She goes out on dates, and I think that anybody would enjoy her company. But this thing about men being attracted to you . . . Maybe she knew something I didn't know.

Life has dealt Beth a double whammy. She's had leukemia since she was eleven, and had a bout with herpes encephalitis, a rare viral infection of the brain, during her early twenties. The herpes encephalitis seemed to go away in about nine months—she says she was very skinny, but she was up and about and walking without a cane by then. However, it seems to have been reactivated in 1985 by the drugs she took for a relapse of the leukemia.

In 1985 she was working in a hospital in Boston, having given up her idea of going to medical school but still having a lot of expertise in biology and statistics, and so on. She worked as a medical statistician.

I called her and we talked. I asked her what she did for romance. The story about her health was undeniably terrible; the story about her love life, though, was pretty much like anybody else's. Few of her lovers (by no means, Phillip, all of them) have disabilities, and some of them were "absolutely gorgeous" and not at all disabled. The normalcy of her experience with men was reassuring.

Even her self-doubt was reassuring—and awfully familiar. She was in a wheelchair by 1986 and by 1987 was involved with a handsome man from where she worked. "I was never gorgeous or anything; just kind of average. David was absolutely gorgeous, and here I am in a wheelchair. I thought, either he's blind, or I can't see what I'm projecting to other people."

Three weeks after they first got together, David and Beth went to Florida. Beth was attending a convention and had to work, but David went primarily to sightsee.

"I felt kind of like a burden. We rented a car and he was driving. He'd drop me off and we'd take apart my wheelchair and then we d put it together again—we had to do that anytime we went anywhere. It was a little bit strained on my part. I just felt nervous. He was fine and calm and didn't care, but I still felt awkward."

It's unlikely that feeling you're a burden is entirely imaginary, though I would like to say so. People with disabilities often try to compensate for this, but unless the time-out is very long, waiting for a disabled person is really no big deal. Beth contrasts her trip with "normal" David with a trip she took with someone she described as "more disabled than I am."

"I went to Chicago with a friend who is a lot more disabled than I am. I had to help him with his chair, get him in the car, et cetera. It was so much work for me; I didn't enjoy the trip at all, though I did get to sightsee a bit. But it was so much work, and I had to wait for him, wait for him, wait for him. . . . I thought, gee, he was to me the way I was to David . . . but in a lesser degree because David and I had a very strong attraction. There was no attraction on my part for this person that would make the trip worth it."

I think that's the crux of it. A disability may indeed make you slower, and some people sometimes are going to be annoyed by that. But if they care about you, the sacrifice will seem small or they'll hardly notice it at all. I think Beth was right when she said that her mutual attraction with David made the waiting around not matter to him; he wanted to be with her, and if he had to wait, he would.

It really wasn't until the man after David that Beth realized that she was attractive because of something she was projecting; David wasn't the only person who responded to it.

"I was still a little insecure with David because I thought, if I ever break up with him no one is ever going to come along and find me attractive again. But then we did break up, and, oh, yeah, I was disappointed, but right away there was Frank. He was a marathoner and a weight lifter so he was really built, but he had been born with one leg. The relationship with him wasn't so special in and of itself, but he was important to my outlook because I realized then that people were responding to something in me. It wasn't that David was so special that he was attracted to me even though I'm in a wheelchair. It's that I'm projecting something that people like. I felt better about the thing with David dissolving. It wasn't him; it was me."

Beth still thinks that she'd rather "date" than get so involved with someone that she wants to get married. She is also still concerned about being a burden. If the perfect person came along, she says, she might consider marriage. But it isn't something she's looking for right now.

When I went home, Richard called.

He's my boyfriend now but he wasn't then. Perhaps it was this phone call that changed my feelings toward him, made me trust him.

But still testing him, I told him I was afraid I repelled people when I limped and was uncoordinated. That's why I sounded so down.

"Moira!" He sounded gratifyingly horrified when I said that. "People don't think that way!"

"Some do," I said.

And some do (like Phillip). But some don't (like Richard, David, others).

Before Richard and I got "tight," I went to the Bronx Zoo with somebody named Tony, who, by the way, did not know I have MS. I had met him at a party. On this, our first "date," we started by fighting about cigarette smoking in the car.

I was self-righteous. I pleaded for our lungs. He pointed out that it was, after all, his car. And so on. Then we got lost, which put us both in better moods.

At last we arrived at the zoo. I had worn purple high-top sneakers, which I thought were really cute. They were a little too snug and were giving me blisters. We climbed a few steps and Tony said, "You're such a poke! Jake [a mutual friend] told me that you walked so fast he could hardly keep up with you in college."

Grrrr.

"That was almost ten years ago and I was never exactly a gazelle," I snapped as I limped over to a park bench and took the inner soles out of my sneakers. I had put them in because I could go farther when there was cushioning in my shoes. Now I slapped the inner soles in my bag. In these cute but tight basketball shoes, they were worse than worthless.

We started to walk around the park. I wanted to walk leisurely from area to area (I was thinking of conserving energy). I even thought it would be nice to sit a while on a bench and watch the giraffes. Tony, on the other hand, thought we ought to zip around. If we hurried we could see (in a blur) all the animals in one day.

Tony kept smoking. It hadn't stunted his growth; he towered above me, which isn't all that easy to do. I reflected upon how he didn't take care of his health, but I did. My sense of inequity grew. We looked at the wild cats. Then:

"Look at the lazy bums on that coach," Tony said as I gazed longingly at the car going around the park. "They won't even walk!" He struck another match.

"Maybe they can't!" I said. "Maybe they're old people, maybe they're cripples! They've got a right to see the animals, too."

Tony broke in, "The coach is just for kids who watch too much TV. It's gross."

Of course, it would have been much easier if I had told Tony the truth about why I wanted to walk slowly when we first arrived at the park. We could have avoided all this. But I didn't.

By this time I was feeling tired and very flinty; Tony was tired and pretty flinty, too. In fact, we didn't like each other at all. We went into the reptile house. DON'T

LEAN AGAINST THE GLASS! the signs on the glass cages warned.

I bet you think I did. I bet you think I leaned against the glass, it shattered, and the torpid snakes energized suddenly and lashed out at Tony, then wound about his legs.

If this were fiction, that's definitely what would have happened in the reptile house. But I am laboring under the constraints of nonfiction. We left the reptile house without incident. It was now late afternoon.

The park was closing. Everybody was going home. Tony looked at the map and said, "The car is parked about here. We walk north."

Shouldn't I have known? Why didn't I ask to see the map?

My thighs were hurting. That's like the first gong of midnight for Cinderella. To me, aching thighs mean I'll be spastic and jerky soon. But we were almost at the car park.

We got to the car park with me trying to hide my growing, but still subtle, symptoms.

"Oh, no!" said Tony. "This isn't it. We'll have to walk back across the park."

"I'm so depressed," I said.

As we walked back, my legs stiffened and I became ungainly. "Why don't you take off those sneaks," Tony said worriedly. "It would be better to walk barefoot if your feet are hurting that much."

"It won't make any difference," I said dully.

In a little while, we found the car. I was so happy to get inside.

Tony hadn't asked, but I knew he was wondering. "I can't talk about it right now," I said. "I'll explain later."

By the time we got to the restaurant, I was okay again. Tony was a gentleman, and as gentlemen are supposed to do, he pretended nothing unusual had happened. We ordered a couple of glasses of wine with our meal and got slightly silly. We actually had fun. The events of the afternoon were never mentioned.

The next day when he called, I explained what he had seen happen.

"I thought it had to be something like that," he said. Pause. "Well, I'm a gambler, so . . . so I'm betting on you."

Here again, though, autobiography does not live up to fiction. In a good story we would have fallen in love. Well, I can't speak for Tony, but I didn't.

Feeling undesirable is hardly an exclusively female problem. Many men who have MS or another debilitating disease find they are unable to have erections and think they can never satisfy a female partner. They avoid sexual encounters or they blame their "failures" on their wives. Fortunately, it really isn't true that there is nothing to be done about impotence; but nothing can be done for those who maintain their silence.

Men often hide their impotence even from themselves because they just can't bear all the negative associations with it. "You're not a man anymore." "You aren't macho." As one man told me, "It tears you apart."

Impotence (an inability to achieve or sustain an erection) is such a common condition that most people know someone affected by it. But they may never have bothered to think about it and may not realize that it could affect a friend of theirs. So "insensitive" remarks abound, making the affected man retreat further and further into "the closet." But the first step in treating the problem is acknowledging it and then deciding what should be done about it.

Not every couple will want to do something about a man's impotence, although there are a number of ways to "help nature" these days. Some men are satisfied by orgasms caused via masturbation or oral-genital contact, and don't care to go through the surgery or injections that could be used to help them maintain erections long enough to have "normal" intercourse. Some women are satisfied by types of sex other than intercourse, so aren't likely to lobby for the implants or injections mentioned.

On the other hand, they may be hesitant to mention their own desires.

Laurie, for example, had a lover whose impotence was caused by diabetes mellitus. She says, "It would have been nice—especially for him—if he could have an erection and we could have 'normal' intercourse. But sometimes I wonder if I'd really prefer it. He spends so much time on me now, enjoying my body and making sure that I receive pleasure. Possibly he's trying to compensate for not having an erection, but I really don't miss it. I would feel bad if he wasn't receiving any pleasure from me, but I really don't think the impotence means that. He seems to get quite excited and though we don't have conventional sex, I think we are both very happy."

Some women do prefer the intimacy of penile-vaginal contact and feel their sex lives are unsatisfactory without it. And some men feel better about themselves and their ability to satisfy the women in their lives if they have can have relatively "normal" sexual relations. People like this should look into Impotents Anonymous, the brainchild of Bruce and Eileen MacKenzie, which holds meetings around the country. (Write to Impotents Anonymous, 119 South Ruth Street, Maryville, TN 37801-3746.) Their advice is to consult a urologist familiar with impotency problems. He can give advice on the type of treatment that is most appropriate—injections or an implant. Be warned, however, that the surgery for an implant is very delicate, and the results have been mixed. It is not recommended for people who simply have "poor" erections, if they're capable of having intercourse. Injections, on the other hand, are recommended for men whose impotence is thought to be potentially reversible. The drugs used might possibly cause liver damage and must be carefully monitored.

All in all, there are many options available; each should be investigated to find out which is right for you. Remember that while sexuality may change because of a disability, it doesn't necessarily have to cease.

10

Sublimating

I am mostly angry, I wrote in my journal a year ago.

Why shouldn't I have been? I wasn't going to run again, or play squash again. Or do lots of the things that I thought were fun. I felt like not doing anything. I felt like just sitting there, so I did for a while. And I cried again.

You need to use these intense and terrible feelings, or else they do something to you. If they aren't used in a creative way, they become destructive. I remember reading *Ethan Frome* and being horrified by the cranky invalid the young woman becomes after her accident. While anyone who has had a serious misfortune deserves to complain a bit, nobody wants to become a chronic complainer, and nobody enjoys a chronic complainer.

Complaining is not the only way to express your feelings—there are lots of productive ways to vent the rage and sadness disability or illness brings. You can vent your feelings about the experience not by complaining nonstop, but by using them to propel you into some meaningful work.

The most successful people use latent abilities, old and neglected or sometimes brand-new ambitions, when for some reason their plans fall through. I spoke to a psychiatrist who put it succinctly. She said, "The most successful people are not afraid to change horses in the middle of a stream."

"But I thought you weren't supposed to do that!" I said.

"Well, you'd better if your horse is dying under you," she said.

Another way to put it: Be flexible. Those "most successful people" are able to change to accommodate unexpected circumstances. They may be ambitious, but the ways they achieve their goals aren't always foreseen.

There's no point in banging your head against a brick wall, which is what I stubbornly did at first. Change. Find a way to work with your problems instead.

If you depend on real or imagined past glory, your current values haven't changed enough to concentrate upon the most admirable abilities still residing within you.

The abilities I've still got—intellectual, artistic—are good ones to have, I think. It would be nice to be smarter and more talented, but at least I still have what I have. These things are more important to me than the physical abilities I've lost. (I still admire physical abilities, of course, and I sure wish I still had them.) But a person in my position must learn to use the abilities she's still got to go forward.

Nancy Fried is someone who moved forward. At forty, Nancy was a vibrant sculptor who seemed active and healthy; at forty-one, she had lost a breast because of cancer. Like anyone confronting a similar situation, she was gripped by anger and fear. Because she had had a mastectomy, in a culture where breasts are supposed to be young and blemish-free forever, she also felt mutilated and sexless.

"Because I am an artist, it was very natural for me to make sculptures of these feelings. In fact, all my work has an autobiographical slant. When I started these sculptures I never expected to show them to anybody." They have, however, become Nancy's most popular work; she's even sold a few pieces to the Metropolitan Museum of Art.

"One of the first pieces I did was of a torso with a screaming head," she says. The face is furious; breasts cascade out of the back of the head. The breasts became a symbol for her—not the typical one of life, maternal love, and satisfaction, but one that women can relate to just as well, although it has the opposite meaning—the fear of death and asexuality; the fear of one's life and sexuality unexpectedly and undeservedly ending.

Nancy's subsequent work—all one-breasted female torsos in her own image—followed her through various stages in her reaction to the disease. One of her later pieces is of a one-breasted woman holding her skirts out on each side the way little girls sometimes do. It's a proud and sexy figure defiantly called "The Flirt." "I did that when I realized that there's life, there's sexuality, after mastectomy.

"When I look at a group of these pieces, the early ones remind me of Brazilian ex-voto figures," she says. (Ex-voto figures are little statues people in Brazil used to make, with oversized parts to indicate "where they hurt." The figure had a huge arm if an arm was injured, or a large head if headaches were the problem. The people would leave the figures in a church, believing that then the injury would be healed.)

Nancy's early work may indeed have been a "plea" on her part for the health and wholeness that has been denied her. And her sculptures do seem to have had a healing effect—according to Nancy, they have definitely helped heal her psyche and possibly have had a positive influence on her physical person, as well. Right now she says she's doing well in many aspects of her life—she seems to be faring well physically, she and her lover are happy together, her work is going well and selling in unexpected amounts.

She thinks that perhaps her recent work moves more people because the anguish and grief it expresses is really universal, one of the dark aspects of the human condition. The work has become far larger in size, indicating that Nancy takes herself seriously and believes her feelings are important. The themes are larger and bolder, too, she says; quite simply, they are loss and regeneration.

In at least one way, however, Nancy's current work is not like the ex-voto figures, because it is celebratory. It celebrates the life and vitality of a woman who has been through a lot.

"Because I was working on the sculptures and looking at the scar frequently, I began to see it not only as normal but as beautiful. This change is reflected in the work—or maybe it is a result of the work which is no longer so much about loss as about life; life which is never perfect, always vulnerable."

Making the statues was a way of "owning" the scar, instead of always feeling frightened and intruded upon by it. "I decided that I couldn't afford to feel ugly and to be ashamed of my body; after all, it's my only body and it's been there through every part of my life," Nancy says. "I don't wear a prosthesis anymore, though many women do to balance themselves. But I found it too uncomfortable, and because I'm large-breasted, it's obvious without it that I've undergone mastectomy. A woman at the market I shop at came up to me and said, 'The first time I saw you I thought—why is she exposing me to that, she has no right! I felt angry at you, but then I thought well, see, it's okay . . . it was such a relief. I've been so terrified of mastectomy.'

"I felt that I had done something for this woman and for the women whom we found crying tears of relief at my last gallery show. The secret was out."

Nancy really believes in "putting the secret out there"—whether it's mastectomy or something else. Feelings that are hidden just fester, she says; but when you uncover them and work with them, you can transform the negative into positive—as she did by making sculptures out of her fear and pain.

Some people want to keep their work to themselves or simply translate it further so that its original source is less obvious. Sometimes it isn't even clear to them why they're doing something that ultimately has the purgative effect Nancy says her work has had on her.

Arthur is a neurobiologist who works on vision research. He is also dyslexic. For most of his life, he was an electrical engineer, but finally " just had to know" more about the brain and vision—the source of dyslexia. He went back to school knowing that, as someone whose reading was labored, he had chosen a tough course of study. He also knew he was "changing horses in the middle of the steam," and that that alone was risky. His work as an electrical engineer was comfortable, but he felt compelled by the neurobiology.

When Arthur returned to school, he was a "grown-up graduate student," already in his forties. By the time he had his Ph.D., he was in his fifties. Now, however, he feels he is involved in personally meaningful work. "The questions I'm addressing in my work concern the visual system but have nothing to do with dyslexia. Still, I'm sure that my feelings about that condition are what makes me want to understand the visual areas in the brain."

Working on the visual system is also a way for Arthur to deal with the frustration caused by dyslexia. The work may not have any particular relevance to the condition, but it's a way of using the emotional energy that the condition evoked in a positive way.

My friend Jane's second daughter, Rachel, was born with optic nerve hypoplasia—a condition in which the optic nerve, which relays visual information to the brain, is underdeveloped. In Rachel's case, only 50 percent is there. She is blind and also has the seizures and mental retardation often associated with the condition.

When Rachel was first diagnosed at two months old, the future looked bleak, and Jane was almost overcome by despair. But eventually she began to find joy and purpose in living again—though this time she had to look for it.

Optic nerve hypoplasia (ONH) is the result of an error in fetal development; no one knows why it happens. At first Rachel was totally blind, although she did acquire some vision when her eyes finished developing, when she was around nine months old. It is still too early to say how much or how useful that vision might be.

Jane had done everything to be healthy during her pregnancy—she was a vegetarian, and even drank only bottled water. She'd had an amniocentesis, although she was only in her early thirties and her husband in his early fifties. It hadn't indicated any problems. This wasn't the child she had expected.

She wondered if, despite her precautions, she had done something to make this happen. Could it have been the running she did during her pregnancy that caused her child to be damaged? But she had run during her first pregnancy, and that daughter was fine. The mothers of other children with Rachel's problem were certainly not all runners, and, besides, doctors had told her it was all right for her to run. But what if it wasn't, what if it was her fault?

In Jane's calmer moments she knew it wasn't her fault. But like most people confronting personal tragedy, she felt disaster might have been averted if only she had done something differently. Even when we know better, most of us feel that, somehow, we're to blame for whatever bad things happen to us.

Jane helped herself by maintaining her involvement in writing and running. These activities let her know that there was more to her life than being the mother of a brain-damaged child. These pursuits "sublimated" her feelings, providing avenues to achievement and self-satisfaction for her; they gave her pleasure and time when she was responsible only for herself, when trying *could* make things better.

When Rachel was first diagnosed, Jane's writing deteriorated; she couldn't concentrate. She tried to write between ten and three as usual, and actually did finish the first draft of her second novel around Rachel's birthday, but working was difficult for her. "Rachel would be lying on a blanket on the floor of my study and I'd keep worrying about her. Without my attention, I thought she was lost in a void."

After submitting her manuscript, Jane began working on a screenplay with her partner, Linda FeFerman. The movie made from their script was released as a feature film and was distributed by Warner Bros. as *Seven Minutes In Heaven*.

As soon as the screenplay left her hands, she started work on a new book, though she could have started the second draft of her novel. But this book had an urgency for her. It is titled *Loving Rachel* and is about her experiences as the mother of a handicapped child.

Writing *Loving Rachel* was healing in some way, Jane says, though she finds it hard to articulate how. She found it emotionally difficult yet compelling: "It was like reliving all those painful moments again." But this time she went over them thoughtfully, knowing that she has accommodated this difficult daughter into her life.

She continues to run, and ran even through the most traumatic periods, about thirty miles a week. Some days she thought she was just too depressed to move, but then found running made her feel better. Running was a familiar part of her routine, and she knew she was good at it. It gave her ballast when life seemed terribly insecure.

During "dark nights" she still worries that Rachel will grow up to be "a strange and lonely person whom no one will love." But for the most part, she thinks of

Rachel as she is now: a cheerful little girl. There will always be heartache involved with having such a child; but despite Rachel's disabilities, Jane loves who she is.

———————

I myself have "sublimated" my feelings in many different ways—by painting, by writing, and by studying neuroscience.

Soon after I learned I have multiple sclerosis, I started my most passionate painting phase. I spread out lots of canvases and squeezed gobs of Winsor-Newton oil paints onto a Saran Wrap palette. I started a series of "broken hearts," which have a nice shape, as well as being evocative. I curled up on the floor and tried to make them de Kooningesque. I'd work like this for hours.

I used both ends of the paint brush, I used cat hair, I used dental floss. I brought in sand and little pieces of glass from the street to embed in the wet paint. They sure weren't realistic paintings. I probably had five canvasses going like this, plus the naked backs of hunched-over women.

How to explain the relief I got from this? Painting is about the most soothing thing I know. I have no real expectations—though I've had paintings in a couple of shows since then, I really don't worry about them having value as something other than self-expression.

Writing about MS was natural to me. I just had to, but not at first. At first, I didn't want to verbalize the feelings. They were still in a wild, inchoate state, and painting was a better medium for me then. However, later I wrote articles about myself and about people with various disabilities, which led to my being approached about writing this book.

Most recently, I've decided to take my interest in neuroscience seriously! I'm back at school. When I first began to read neuroscience, I was frustrated (and furious) that there is no known cure for MS. As I said earlier, I began to read neurology textbooks, certain that the cure was there just waiting to be recognized. Of course, even though I read every line with passionate attention, I didn't find that elusive cure. I found something else, though—a fascination with neuroscience. Five years after my first encounter with it, I've resolved to spend a large part of my life studying and researching the brain.

Most people are fascinated by any disease or injury they have. I'm no different. But I think my interest in neuroscience goes beyond the curiosity and the fallacious control-it-by-knowing-about-it feeling engendered by having MS. I wasn't sure about my motives at first, so I gave myself some pretty dry studying to do—mostly in neuroanatomy—to see if I could "hack it" and prove my commitment. I have; I love neuroscience. My emotional response to having MS probably propels my studies somewhat, but it isn't the only thing propelling them.

Although MS introduced me to neuroscience, I don't concentrate on reading about demyelinating disorders with mostly physical symptoms. It's too upsetting. Besides, good minds, less biased and better equipped than mine, are working hard to stop these illnesses. Instead, I'm interested in cognitive and affective disorders such as schizophrenia. Again, there's a personal interest here: One of my good friends in college became severely schizophrenic after I graduated. Although I still see her occasionally, she has become one of the "living dead." What happened?

I would like to earn a Ph.D. in neuropsychology and do research on schizophrenia. This kind of work seems important, necessary, and enthralling to me. I think my own experience with a neurological disorder (albeit a very different one from schizophrenia) has taught me the limits of willpower in trying to deal with the brain gone wrong. It can only add urgency to the search for understanding and intervention.

I know other people who have used their energies in new ways because of a debilitating disease. Peter has a rare, congenital neuromuscular condition called congenital spinal muscular atrophy, and has used a wheelchair since he was a child. It is not a degenerative disease and has "reasonably stabilized," although, he says, "some fairly unpleasant things" are likely to happen in the future. He is now thirty years old and can't walk at all. But Peter is a very intelligent and perceptive thinker. He uses his mental abilities to think of ways to improve his life and the lives of other disabled people.

Peter doesn't actually "sublimate" his feelings about being disabled the way Nancy and Jane use their feelings in their respective arts; but, like them, he uses his abilities—in his case, a facility with legal codes and an understanding of government—to help himself and others like him. He is more like Arthur, the neurobiologist with dyslexia, because he uses his intellectual abilities to relieve the frustration caused by his disabling condition. In Arthur's case, though, the work is his vocation; in Peter's case, the work is an avocation and not his main source of livelihood.

Peter is a lawyer who attended a major university law school. While there, he delved into the laws of the state and put together a catalog of every regulation and code that referred to disabled people—for example, what kind of facilities and services should be available for them in various public places and institutions—and organized a group of students to take appropriate legal action when they found shortfalls. He continues to compile the legal obligations a place has, and teaches other handicapped people how to get action by taking legal measures when the obligations are not fulfilled and their needs are not met. Peter says this type of work is both useful and satisfying to him.

Peter is a practical man, and disability isn't new to him. Nevertheless, it requires many tasks of him that he still considers onerous. For example, law is not his first love; statecraft is. Peter has loved public affairs since he was in high school, and he has an advanced degree from the Woodrow Wilson School at Princeton University. But as an assistant professor of public affairs, he was not able to earn enough money to take care of himself. Peter needs to hire attendants; he needs to have a van to transport him and his wheelchair. The costs of transit and living space are much more for him than they are for a normal person; in fact, his living expenses are about twice what the average person's are, just for necessities.

As a lawyer, concentrating on fairly lucrative areas, Peter can care for himself financially. He enjoys law, but it is primarily "a vehicle of independence" for him.

Peter's feelings of anger—certainly appropriate in his condition—have found an outlet in his legal work for the handicapped. The work itself may be strictly intellectual and rational, but his personal and emotional interest in a case brought against an institution that is not fulfilling its legal obligations must be a factor in the time and effort he spends on the enterprise. Work like this is both useful to other people and a healthy relief for oneself.

I went to a meeting of the Networking Project, a group of disabled professional women who wanted to act as role models for disabled teenage girls. One of the women I met was a neurochemist named Lynn. She had an interpreter with her because she had been deaf from meningitis since age eleven.

Lynn was about fifty, blonde and attractive. At first I spoke to her very loudly. ("Nice weather we're having!" I shouted.) But it made no difference to her whether or not I spoke at the top of my lungs, and I began to feel sheepish. I started speaking to her in a normal voice when I realized that that was what everyone else was doing. At least, I told myself, I hadn't been exaggeratedly mouthing the words. That's what many people do when they talk to someone who is reading their lips, and they just make it harder.

Lots of faux pas are easy to make when dealing with people who are missing different abilities. As a normal person you have to forget about the discomfort misunderstanding disabilities causes *you*. You can only try to be sensitive and do the right thing. It's inevitable that even with the best intentions, you'll make mistakes; but you're probably not the first person to make them. Your mistakes, even your prejudices, probably come from lack of exposure.

Lynn was an excellent lip-reader. If she could watch your face while you were talking, the two of you could carry on a conversation with little problem. Her voice was a little strange—high, not normally modulated, childish, and unusually sweet. Having been able to hear speech in the past helped her use her voice fairly "normally."

She rarely used her interpreter. He took over when several people were talking at once and gave her the gist of what they were saying. He was very smooth in deciding when she needed him and when to leave her alone. I faced her (at last I was getting the hang of it) and said I'd come to her office the following week.

The next week I took a bus to the medical center where Lynn worked. Her secretary showed me into her office. I asked her questions about living with deafness. She told me that her doorbell showed that it had been rung by turning on a light bulb in her apartment; her life was made easier by practical things like that.

She also talked about her years in school. She used to go to lectures even though she couldn't hear her professors, and when they turned toward the blackboards, she couldn't even read their lips. But so much happens at a lecture that isn't in the books. Though she'd been told by a dean that she could skip the lectures, she wanted to be at them. If she couldn't understand what was happening, she'd just ask another student.

After graduating from college, she worked for years as a lab technician. This was boring, she said. It took the women's movement to allow her to picture herself as a scientist. She had never heard of a deaf female scientist, but eventually she decided to go back to school at night. Voilá! Soon she was here, and she loved her work.

Lynn said her way of "sublimating" was working with the disabled teenage girls in the Networking Project. She thought it was very important for them to know that being a scientist was not an impossible dream. Disabled people who are scientifically inclined can work in a lab— it's not necessary to become a scientist, she added. Whatever a disabled person did in a lab would depend partly on the disability, of course. A person in a wheelchair could work very well with a microscope. A blind person would naturally do something else.

Working with others who share some of your problems and concerns, like Lynn does with the teenage girls and Peter does with the disabled people and the law, is a great way to use your special experience to help other people. And helping other people is one of the most satisfying things that anyone can do.

Another way of sublimating can be through religious faith. I asked the monseigneur in the local church some questions about illness and faith. "The reason for human suffering is a mystery," said the monseigneur. "But faith in a God who allows suffering but doesn't cause it is the most strengthening thing I know. People who reach out to God are soothed, and survive without becoming bitter and sullen."

I went through eight years of Catholic grammar school. I went to Catholic high school, too. Faith is famous for raising, or eliminating, one's threshold of despair. It seems to help people who have nowhere left to turn. And the recuperative power of faith is noted again and again by both psychologists and people who work in rehabilitation medicine. I thought somewhere in my heart of hearts I must believe. And now, Griffin (I said to myself), it looks like it would really behoove you to believe.

Granted, there's something very unappealing about "deathbed conversions," but I think all the "faithful," as believers were always called when I was in school, are driven by need. In any case, I wasn't too proud: If religion would give me solace, I would humbly accept it. I started trying to understand faith. I tried to find faith in me.

"Human brokenness only increases when one feels isolated and as if no one cares. When you have faith, you are never alone," the monseigneur explained to me.

There's no question that faith helps people cope. Psychologists often recommend that people lean on existing ties and consider looking into the religion in which they were raised when they are confronted with a serious situation. Even my neurologist mentioned religion to me twice.

Faith seemed to have much to do with the recovery of Brigitte Gerney, who received national attention in 1985 when she was pinned under a fallen crane for five hours in a New York City construction site accident. She prayed with her rescuers as they worked to free her from the wreckage. Gerney had had other traumas in her life, including the death of a child and a personal struggle with cancer. But she maintained faith that her God would watch over her. Gerney's recovery and spirits were reportedly remarkable. The debilitating anger and fear that might have afflicted someone else seemed not to take their toll on her.

When I was a child, I remember a book about the Littlest Angel. He gave Jesus a gift of things from earth— a broken robin's egg, some pebbles—he had left in a box under the bed he had when he was just another human child. In those days, this was my favorite book. And I remember a line from a Kennedy speech: God's work on earth must truly be our own.

I have faith that people are going to find the answer to this and other obnoxious human diseases. As far as a Supreme Being—I'm not sure. I'm a pretty serious person; if I become a believer mine will be a thoughtful and serious faith. Right now it's not part of my make-up. But faith has been so powerful a healing force in so many people's lives that it would be remiss not to mention it.

If you do have faith, cherish it. Think of it as a healing gift. It may be your strongest asset.

What's important is to believe that out of everything—even trouble—comes something worthwhile. Many of us no longer have faith in a conventional religion. But finding personal meaning in whatever happens both enriches your life and makes bad things bearable.

11

Research

The other day I did something I haven't done in ages: I opened a textbook on multiple sclerosis. This was different from the books on neuropsychology that I now diligently study; this book was only about my disease. It was blunt; it didn't care that I was reading it; it didn't mince words. It was detailed and relentless. Suffice it to say that I scared myself again. Once again I whirled in that awful vortex, believing just what was in the book, believing it was right when it stated that someone with my initial symptom was clean out of luck. According to the book, ataxia (what I call wobbling) had the worst prognosis of any MS symptom. Terrible things were in store, and total cripplehood was just around the corner.

I'm sorry MS happened to me. I'm sorry it happens to anyone. But it's five years since I was diagnosed. The textbook must be wrong. I'm about the same as I was when I first was diagnosed—if at all, only a little worse. But according to the textbook, by now I should be in serious trouble. Always check the copyright date on any book about MS—after that text, I refuse to look at anything more than a few years old. Books that are older are likely to be very alarming. Current material makes room for exceptions. Anybody should remember that he or she might be the exception. You have to be reasonable in your expectations, though, unless you want to be disappointed—alas, this is not a disease that really goes away.

I haven't gotten used to MS. However, I'm pretty sure that serious disability is not around the corner for me or for many other people like me. Only 25 percent or so of people diagnosed with MS ever need wheelchairs. So why worry about that? And readers of this book should remember that many people with MS are not as affected as I am. Good for them (the people with very mild cases). I hope they stay that way; a good percentage of them will. (See below for predictions on average rate of worsening.)

I'm often unsteady on my feet. I lurch and stagger every so often, and I wonder what people think. MS has changed my life in negative ways, and I would like more than anything to get better. But the disease has been stable for a long time and it will probably be stable much longer. Believe it or not, I'm glad I've had this experience. (Well, okay, I'm sort of glad.)

Having MS has not conferred sainthood on me or made me courageous or anything like that. But it has taught me some invaluable things. I have more compassion for people who are very disabled than I knew I had in me; I guess because I identify with them in a new way. With all the testimonials about positive attitudes, you'd think you could overcome almost anything if you have the right attitude: The sick should just *will* themselves well. Sorry, but if it was that easy, there'd be a lot less illness in the world and well-loved children would never die.

But well-loved children do die, and people with good attitudes do get ill. There's a lot of evil loose in the universe and, as Harold S. Kushner says, sometimes bad things happen to good people. I've known some very sick people, but I've never known one who *wanted* to be sick—for manipulative purposes, or any others. I suppose such people exist. Nevertheless, if anyone thinks that those unlucky enough to get a disease lack a good enough attitude to stay well, they should think again.

It's bad enough to have a disease without feeling you're to blame for it, too. But I have felt that way and many other people tell me that they have felt that way, too, ashamed of being ill or disabled in some way. As if life wasn't tough enough already.

I admit, though, that nothing beats trying. There's a lot of medical evidence that says a fighting spirit is the healthiest thing around and that psychological well-being does make a difference in a person's health. But I believe there are limits to willpower with a brain gone wrong. I don't think I have a better attitude than people who are sicker than I am—or a worse attitude than the very well.

Because of my own experiences, I think I understand the anger of the very disabled, the very ill; it doesn't remotely scare me. I'm angry even though my disabilities aren't severe—and it makes me understand that kind of anger a little better. It isn't directed at me, anyhow; it's directed at life, which has been so unfair. It seems to be the most human of emotions—outrage that life isn't fair.

I'm still angry. But anger isn't always a damaging thing. Anger can be energizing; it can help you make a difference. I'm using my anger to do things that make that difference.

The night I read that textbook, I cried myself to sleep again—I doubt for the last time. The next morning I said to myself, "Well, you haven't gotten worse, and there are lots of more terrible things that could have happened, so stop feeling sorry for yourself and get on with it, Child." (When I'm mothering myself I call myself Child. Child is a way of gentling what I say because I'm a stern mother. Self-sympathy is good but self-pity is paralyzing, and, alas, it is powerfully seductive.)

I went to work. During lunch hour I went to a nearby library and got out the August 13, 1987, issue of the *New*

England Journal of Medicine (NEJM) as well as the July 1988 issue of *Neurology*. I made a copy of a commonly used Disability Status Scale (DSS)—a standard of assessing neurological deficits. Where did I stand? How about my friend Holly?

The following is an abbreviated form of the Kurtzke Scale:

The DSS or Kurtzke Scale

0—Normal neurological examination
1—No disability and minimal signs during neurological examination
2—Minimal disability: slight weakness OR slight incoordination OR some loss of sensation or vision, etc.
3—Moderate disability though walking independently
4—Relatively severe disability in one of the areas mentioned in 2
5—Walking unaided no more than several blocks
6—Cane, crutch, or brace required to walk 100 m
7—Wheelchair most of the time
8—Bed-bound but with effective use of arms
9—Helpless bed patient
10—Death from MS

What really worries me, though, is what's to come. The MS Society has an average rate of progession for 170 patients at one clinic, which provides you with a good idea of what happens to most MS people—but, of course, any individual might progress more quickly or slowly than the average.

DSS AT FIRST EXAM	NO. OF PATIENTS	DSS 5 YEARS LATER
0	10	0.6
1	22	2.3
2	19	3.4
3	18	4.1

Dss at First Exam	No. of Patients	Dss 5 Years Later
4	14	5.2
5	12	5.8
6	32	6.5
7	28	7.7
8	9	8.3
9	6	9.2

It's still impossible to predict the course of any individuals' MS, but, according to doctors at the MS Society, if several years pass since diagnosis without a significant disability, one can expect a milder course in the future.

A slow progression, though, is not enough to satisfy anybody. We all want to be cured, to be normal again. Many tests are being made, but medical research hasn't found the answer yet.

According to the *NEJM*, "the ultimate goal in the treatment of multiple sclerosis and other autoimmune diseases is to remove or suppress only antigen-specific autoreactive cells." Since myelin basic protein, a major component of myelin, produces experimental autoimmune encephalomyelitis (EAE), the working animal model of multiple sclerosis, many think that it may be very involved in the pathogenesis of MS. However, many other scientists would not agree.

Even in the absence of an agreed-upon antigen, many clinical trials are now under way to (1) effectively treat exacerbations of the disease, (2) prevent or modify future exacerbations, (3) treat the progessive stage, and (4) restore or improve neurological function in apparently stable cases. (See *Therapeutic Claims in Multiple Sclerosis*, 2nd edition, written by members of the Therapeutic Claims Committee of the International Federation of Multiple Sclerosis Societies, for a very complete run-down of the various therapies being tried in MS, written in layperson's language.)

In the January 27, 1989 issue of *Nature*, one of the world's most prestigious science journals, an article appeared which described finding traces of HTLV-1, a retrovirus, in the blood of six Swedish MS patients. If this finding holds up and can be repeated by other scientists working with other MS patients, the information may lead to really effective treatments for the disease. Of course, if HTLV-1 or a retrovirus similar to it is found to be intimately associated with MS, it would not mean that MS is not an autoimmune disease. A virus or retrovirus may simply be the trigger for an autoimmune response.

Treatments currently being tried for MS include:

COP-1

Cop-1 is a mixture of synthetic polymers simulating fragments of myelin basic protein. It does not induce EAE in experimental animals, but instead suppresses it. An article in the *NEJM*, states that studies in animals suggested that cop-1 may work by producing antigen-specific suppressor T cells. Cop-1 was tried in humans and found to have few undesirable side reactions and to be promising—particularly in people with milder forms of the disease. A pilot trial of fifty exacerbating-remitting patients was begun.

During the two years of the pilot trial with exacerbating-remitting patients, (those who have discrete episodes of worsening—exacerbations—and then improve or go into remission), more than half of the twenty-five people who had entered the study and received the cop-1 instead of the placebo (an inert substance) had no exacerbations. The trial was double-blind, so neither the patients nor the researchers knew who was receiving the placebo and who was receiving the real thing. When the code was broken at the end of the study, the results looked good for the patients using the real thing—the cop-1.

Before the trial, all the patients had experienced

about two exacerbations per year. During the study, the placebo group (which ended as only twenty-three people because of two drop-outs) experienced an apparent reduction in rate of exacerbations—but less than half as great as the one experienced by the people on cop-1. So even if the mysterious placebo effect had reduced the rate of exacerbations, it alone could not account for the entire reduction experienced by the people on cop-1.

Less disabled patients (0 to 2 on the Kurtzke Disability Status Scale) improved slightly on cop-1 during the two years—an average of 0.5 on the Kurtzke Scale. This improvement only happened to the group of thirteen patients who started off with less neurological disability. It seems cop-1 was most effective on people whose disease was least advanced. Even their improvement wasn't very great, but still. You can imagine how happy I felt. I felt happy for everybody.

Some time after the successful E-R trial, a trial was begun of cop-1 on chronic-progressive (C-P) MS patients. One hundred six people with the rather serious form of MS called chronic-progressive gave themselves an injection of cop-one or a placebo twice daily during the course of two years. The study was once again double-blinded, so neither the patients nor the doctors knew which substance—the cop-1 or the inert placebo—the patient was receiving.

The amount of cop-1 was greater in this study—15 mg twice a day instead of the 20 mg once a day injected by patients in the previous study. It was completed in the fall of 1988. In November, when most of the results were tabulated, they showed (a) a higher-than-expected response to the placebo; (b) no statistically significant difference between the placebo group and the people really taking cop-1.

The trial is not likely to be rerun, but at the time of this writing that was not decided. Perhaps symptoms that weren't being measured in the study—which concentrated on ability to walk—were being favorably affected. Because symptoms other than walking were possibly being affected by the cop-1, another study might be warranted.

4-AMINOPYRIDINE

An exciting symptomatic treatment (that is, one that doesn't alter the underlying disease process but improves function) is 4-aminopyridine. It blocks potassium channels in the nerve fiber that enhances the current flow through demyelinated areas.

Nerve impulses are dependent on sodium and potassium channels. The sodium channels are concentrated at the nodes of Ranvier, which are the areas that are devoid of myelin and are between the links of a nerve fiber. (Think of the nerve fiber as a long chain of linked sausages. The nodes occur at the places between the sausages.) Potassium channels, conversely, are concentrated in the internodes (or the sausage parts of the chain). They are usually covered up by myelin. When the potassium channels are uncovered, the nerve no longer can conduct impulses. 4-aminopyridine blocks those uncovered potassium channels.

The drug can be administered intravenously or orally. After receiving a dose of 4-aminopyridine, some patients who could not walk without the use of canes or walkers were able to walk for short distances without them. The effects were short-lived, however—only a few hours. The greatest trouble with the drug had become apparent earlier when it was tried in higher doses on myasthenia gravis patients in England: It caused seizures.

Since the drug is not specific to demyelinated patches on the nerve fibers, it increases the activity level of the entire brain. This is what leads to the seizures. A variant of the drug, called 3,4-di aminopyridine, seems to be "attracted" to demyelinated patches and will possibly circumvent this problem. It is being developed now. I certainly hope this drug is successful, even if its effect remains short-lived—imagine having a hiatus of even a few hours every day!—but something will still be needed to stop the disease process itself.

INTERFERONS

Interferon is a substance derived from cells exposed to virus. It interferes with the ability of new cells to help new virus replicate. Interferon was originally thought to be only an antiviral substance, but later it was found to have other properties as well. Because of its antiviral and immunomodulating actions, it might be useful in treating MS.

There are three basic types of interferon—alpha, beta, and gamma. An experiment in which beta interferon was injected directly into the spinal cord of MS patients resulted in fewer exacerbations for those patients—possibly because interferon's antiviral action cut down on the numbers of viral infections that might trigger exacerbations.

Systemic administration (not into the spinal cord but injected into the bloodstream or taken orally) of interferon is preferable because: (1) of the inconvenience of the spinal cord route; (2) of the fact that immune functions outside the central nervous system show some abnormalities in MS patients; and (3) it avoids the risks associated with spinal cord administration. One of the questions a trial of interferon treatment might address is whether it should be administered just during exacerbations or whether treatment should be continuous.

The gamma interferon trial, which had a negative effect, may actually have been a blessing in disguise for MS patients. Gamma interferon intensifies the immune response. It was administered to MS patients on the theory that it might have antiviral properties or affect immunity in a positive way, but it just made the disease more voracious and the study patients suffered additional exacerbations. They recovered "reasonably well," say their doctors, and no one with MS will be given gamma interferon in the future. But it did present researchers with a new plan of attack, which is currently under investigation: diminishing the effect of naturally produced gamma interferon in MS patients.

These experiments may only be a "foot in the door" right now, but they represent a good start.

MONOCLONAL ANTIBODIES

Monoclonal (single) antibodies are an exciting potential treatment because they seem to be very specific. In other words, they might be able to augment or suppress the immune response in one specific area without affecting areas that seem to be doing just fine. This means that the risk of getting other diseases as a result of the treatment for one disease will be enormously reduced. This is the "magic bullet" specificity: It is described by the MS Society as similar to a rifle that shoots a single bullet right at its target. Other less specific drugs are more like shotguns that spray bullets all over and probably hit their targets, but a lot of other things as well.

Knocking out the immune system in a person with an autoimmune disease is not a good idea. Although the overactive immune system may no longer be a problem, the person will then be vulnerable to all sorts of other diseases. Monoclonal antibodies may circumvent this problem by acting only on the parts of the immune system that are overactive in an autoimmune disease.

At this point, the major drawback to this potential therapy is that people develop antibodies against the monoclonal antibodies. The original monoclonal antibodies tried on people with MS were produced in mice. With repeated infusions, however, people produced anti-mouse antibodies, rendering the treatment ineffective. Newer, suppressive monoclonal antibodies will, hopefully, be accepted by human beings, eliminating this problem. Someday they may even be used to halt the MS process. This treatment is still experimental, of course, and is very expensive.

PLASMAPHERESIS

Plasmapheresis is a procedure in which blood is taken from the patient and put through an apheresis machine to separate the plasma and cell parts. Then the plasma part, thought to contain antibodies and other substances that damage myelin and slow nerve conduction—such as serum immunoglobulins, myelin basic protein, and immune complexes—is discarded and replaced by albumin and normal human plasma. The reconstituted whole blood is put back in the patient.

At the same time, the patient is on an immunosuppressive drug regimen. Immunosuppressive drugs seem to prevent the "rebound" effect in which the bloodstream refills with the material that's been removed.

According to the MS Society, plasmapheresis is still a highly experimental treatment with conflicting results in controlled trials. The procedure is very expensive, costing $500 to $800 for each exchange—and the exchanges must be done every few days or weeks. Plasmapheresis is, however, relatively free of adverse side effects, and some investigators are excited by the fact that it seems to affect very disabled MS patients who are otherwise resistant to therapy.

CYCLOPHOSPHAMIDE OR CYTOXAN

Cyclophosphamide is an immunosuppressant drug developed as a cancer treatment. It has been tested only on patients who have a rapidly progessive form of the disease because the side effects associated with its use do not warrant its administration to anyone less severely affected.

There have been conflicting reports regarding the drug's efficacy, and the side effects include hair loss and nausea. It is considered an investigational drug whose use at this point is restricted to the very ill.

COLCHICINE

Colchicine is a commonly used antigout drug that has both antiinflammatory and immunosuppressant properties. This is a potentially beneficial treatment for MS, although a trial testing its usefulness has not yet been concluded. Its side effects, however, include diarrhea severe enough to be a serious drawback to its long-term use. There are also possibly serious long-term effects. It is easily available, however, and not costly, which might be strong recommendations for it if it proves to be useful in MS.

STEROIDS

Most MS patients experience an acute attack—an exacerbation—at some time, and they will probably be prescribed a course of steroid treatment. Steroids shorten an acute attack by about 10 percent—it's thought by reducing the inflammation surrounding the demyelinated nerve fiber. In the long run, however, steroids do not seem to be effective in altering the course of MS, although they may be useful in conjunction with some other therapy. ACTH, Solu Medrol, prednisone are the names of some of the steroids commonly used.

IMURAN

Imuran, or azathioprine, is an immunosuppressant drug that may slow the progression of disability in people who are severely affected by MS. There is no rigorous evidence that it does so, however, but risks associated with its use (non-Hodgkins' lymphoma, other cancers) may be acceptable when the risks of severe disability caused by MS are greater. Proof of efficacy is not available, but some experienced physicians claim that their patients on the drug do better than their patients who are not. Lacking powerful evidence one way or the other yet, it is up to the discretion of the physician and his or her patient to decide whether or not use of this drug is warranted.

TOTAL LYMPHOID IRRADIATION

Lymph nodes all over the body are X-rayed daily for about six weeks in this immunosuppressant treatment. One study in New Jersey showed TLI slowed the deterioration of chronic progressive multiple sclerosis. The benefits have been seen to last at least four years. The benefits are greatest for those who show the greatest degree of lymphopenia (lymphocytes are responsible for tissue destruction in autoimmune disease) immediately after treatment. The costs are high, and it is still an experimental treatment. Modification of the treatment to benefit more patients is being studied.

THC

When I was a kid, I would have loved this treatment. Maybe I've become stuffy in my old age, but the mind-altering effects of this drug are its biggest drawback to me. Oh, and, yes, there's the fact that it's illegal.

Some people say that marijuana or its active ingredient, tetrahydrocannabinol (THC), reduces their spasticity. *Science News* reports that preliminary studies show that, indeed, THC may work quickly and effectively during severe episodes. It may also suppress the immune system, and it is not known to have serious side effects. However, memory deficits may be associated with it.

ESSENTIAL FATTY ACIDS (EFA)

Prostaglandins, which are known to modify immune response, can be increased by administration of their precursor substances, essential fatty acids. Analysis of three double-blind controlled trials of EFA has shown that those patients having only minimal or no disability at entry into the trial had a significantly smaller increase in disability and a lower exacerbation rate than comparable placebo patients.

EFAs are effective, but their effects are modest. In the form of Evening Primrose Oil they can be bought at any health food store, and in sunflower seed and safflower seed oil they can be used as salad dressings. Fish oils—as in cod liver oil and others—also seem to have a modest benefit and are readily available.

This treatment appears to be medically sound but to have only modest (but real) benefits.

The research being done right now is exciting and promising. I feel sure that an end to the ravages of MS and at least some restoration of function will be possible in the foreseeable future. I don't allow myself to be too sanguine, however, because, like anybody else with MS, I've been disappointed in the past when promising-looking leads turned out to be dead ends. But I still believe in staying ready for good news. Everyone—and especially anyone with a slowly progressive disease such as MS usually is—should keep as healthy as possible so he or she can reap all the benefits that good health and long life will bring. I believe in doing this because someday I *am* going to be cured, and so are you.

Sources and background for therapies mentioned in Chapter 11 that are currently being researched include:

Bornstein, M., et al. "A Pilot Trial of Cop-1 in Exacer-bating-Remitting Multiple Sclerosis." *New England Journal of Medicine* (Aug. 13, 1987).

Interviews with M. Bornstein and V. Spada on cop-1 trials.

Interview with S. Reingold on general research issues.

Kurtzke, J. F. "Rating Neurological Impairment in Multiple Sclerosis: An Expanded Disability Status Scale." *Neurology* 33 (1983): 1444.

Mertin, J. "Drug Treatment of Patients with Multiple Sclerosis." in *Demyelinating Diseases*, ed. Johan C. Koetsier. Handbook of Cliniical Neurology, Vol. 47, 3rd ed. New York, Elsevier Science Publishing Company, 1985.

"Multiple Sclerosis Update: A Symposium." *Neurology* 30: 1, 1980.

"Rationale for Immunomodulating Therapies of Multiple Sclerosis: A Symposium." *Neurology* 38: 2 (1988).

Sibley, William A., and the Therapeutic Claims Committee of the International Federation of Multiple Sclerosis Societies, eds. *Therapeutic Claims in Multiple Sclerosis*, 2d ed. New York: Demos Publications, 1988.

Epilogue

Going the Distance

When I first began to write this book, I thought only about going the distance physically. I realized that I could not run or walk the way I had before MS became symptomatic, but I thought it was important to cover the same ground any old which way I could—to "go the distance."

Now going the distance physically is (almost) the last thing I think about. Of course, going the distance physically would still be pleasant and convenient, and doing it "normally" would be inexpressibly sweet. But I want to do other things even more: I want to go the distance intellectually and emotionally now. In other words, I want to use every scrap of intelligence I've got and every emotion I've felt—especially the anguish I've felt because of MS—to make a difference to the people who read this book. Just by understanding and allowing their anger, I think I can make an emotional difference there.

I guess I've become awfully serious. (Well, this has been a sobering experience.) Not that I don't laugh anymore—I do, every chance that I get—but I think about life as a rather serious undertaking now. I've changed

147

horses in the middle of the stream, and now I'm concentrating on learning about nervous system diseases that affect the ability to think and feel. This scientific stuff I totally ignored as an English major, but I just can't imagine anything that's as important as neuropsychology now, since it contributes to the understanding and eradication of these illnesses.

But my own neurological disease may very well put a cramp in my ambitions in neuropsychology. MS sometimes does cause cognitive deficits. This worries me more than the physical impositions it causes; it's not likely to cause severe deficits in mentation like Alzheimer's Disease does, but even a minor deficit might mean I'll have to change horses again. It's excruciating to think that you might be losing your smarts and there's nothing you can do to stop it. I haven't seen any evidence of it happening, though, and I'm not going to plan on it. I'm going to count on being cured, but I *will* make a contingency plan.

I was in the hospital once, having a course of steroids that didn't help the MS at all (oh well, the steroids were worth trying). I met lots of people with neurological disorders—many of which included deficits in mentation. I felt no comfort in being better off than the other patients there; I simply felt an urgency to see an end to some of these diseases in my lifetime.

This is an exciting time in MS research because real progress is being made. But the cure isn't here yet, and I don't want to wait for it—I want every moment to be worthwhile. I want to deal with MS a little more gracefully than I have in the past; I want to use what intelligence I have (and be grateful for it, though it isn't as much as I'd like) to do work that matters. I want to make life more bearable for people it's been especially unkind to. I've decided I can do that, by allowing them to be as angry and miserable around me as anybody experiencing a misfortune has a right to be. I know how unusual it is to find someone who allows you to "not be nice" but angry. And to, hopefully, do research that will help people with neuropsychological disorders. I also want to ensure that

I'll never be a financial or emotional burden to the people I love. This is actually quite a hefty agenda.

There are many ways to go the distance. While I'm busy going the distance in these nonphysical ways, I feel sure that effective treatments and a real cure for MS will be developed.

I hope you decide to go the distance, too.

Further Reading

The following books have been very helpful to me at different times. They represent a rather wide and idiosyncratic approach to dealing with a chronic illness. Sometimes they are scientific and rational, sometimes they deal with disease as it's experienced and can be easily understood by the layperson, and sometimes they are spiritual and/or emotional guides.

I include, too, Jane Bernstein's book about being the mother of a mentally and visually disabled child because I think it's instructive to see how grieving is so similar, when the cause is so different.

But all these books deal with living well. Take a look at some of them—they may help you, too.

BERNSTEIN, JANE. *Loving Rachel*. Boston: Little, Brown and Company, 1988.

COLLIGAN, DOUGLAS, and LOCKE, STEPHEN, M.D. *The Healer Within*. New York: E. P. Dutton, 1986.

COUSINS, NORMAN. *Anatomy of an Illness*. New York: W. W. Norton, 1979.

KLEINMAN, ARTHUR, M. D. *The Illness Narratives*. New York: Basic Books, 1988.

KUSHNER, HAROLD. *When Bad Things Happen to Good People*. New York: Avon Books, 1981.

LECHTENBERG, RICHARD, M.D. *Multiple Sclerosis Fact Book*. Philadelphia: F.A. Davis Company.

LEMAISTRE, JOANNE. *Beyond Rage*. Oak Part, IL: An Alpine Guild Book, 1985.

MAIRE, NANCY. *Plaintext*. Tucson: University of Arizona Press, 1987.

MATTHEWS, W. B., et al. *McAlpine's Multiple Sclerosis*. New York: Churchill Livingstone, 1985.

ROSNER, LOUIS J., M.D., and ROSS, SHELLEY. *Multiple Sclerosis*. New York: Prentice-Hall Press, a Division of Simon & Schuster, Inc., 1987.

SCHEINBERG, LABE, M.D. *Multiple Sclerosis: A Guide for Patients and Their Families*, 2d ed. New York: Raven Press, 1987.

SHUMAN, ROBERT, and SCHWARTZ, JANICE. *Understanding Multiple Sclerosis*. New York: Charles Scribner's Sons, 1988.

SONTAG, SUSAN. *Illness as Metaphor*, New York: Farrar Straus Giroux, 1978.